Liver and Biliary Surgery

Handbooks in General Surgery

Kirby I. Bland • Michael G. Sarr
Markus W. Büchler • Attila Csendes
O. James Garden • John Wong
Editors

Liver and Biliary Surgery

Handbooks in General Surgery

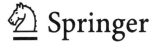 Springer

Editors

Kirby I. Bland, MD
Fay Fletcher Kerner Professor
and Chairman
Department of Surgery
Deputy Director
Comprehensive Cancer Center
University of Alabama School
of Medicine
Birmingham, AL, USA

Michael G. Sarr, MD
James C. Mason Professor
of Surgery
Department of Surgery
Mayo Clinic College of
Medicine
Rochester, MN, USA
sarr.michael@mayo.edu

Markus W. Büchler, MD
Professor of Surgery
and Chairman
Department of General
and Visceral Surgery
University of Heidelberg
Heidelberg, Germany
markus_buechler@med.
uni-heidelberg.de

Attila Csendes, MD, FACS
(Hon)
Professor of Surgery
and Chairman
Department of Surgery
University Hospital
Santiago, Chile
acsendes@machi.med.uchile.cl

O. James Garden, MBChB, MD,
FRCS (Ed), FRCP (Ed),
FRACS (Hon)
Regius Professor of Clinical
Surgery
Department of Clinical
and Surgical Sciences
The University of Edinburgh
Royal Infirmary of Edinburgh
Edinburgh, UK
Email: o.j.garden@ed.ac.uk

John Wong, BSc (Med (Syd)),
MBBS (Syd),
PhD (Syd), MD
(Hon (Syd)),
FRACS, FRCS (Edin),
FRCS (Glasg), FACS (Hon)
Chair Professor
Department of Surgery
The University of Hong Kong
Queen Mary Hospital
Hong Kong, China

ISBN 978-1-84996-428-9   e-ISBN 978-1-84996-429-6

DOI 10.1007/978-1-84996-429-6

Springer Dordrecht Heidelberg London New York

British Library Cataloguing in Publication Data

A catalogue record for this book is available from the British
Library

Library of Congress Control Number: 2010938113

Printed on acid-free paper

Springer is part of Springer Science+Business Media (www.springer.com)

Preface

The editors designed the original textbook, *General Surgery: Principles and International Practice* from which this shorter paperback monograph on liver and biliary surgery was taken to be an accessible, concise, and state-of-the-art volume that explores and documents evolutionary principles in the practice of surgery. This work is aimed at the general surgeon and the resident in training. The scientific community continues to witness extraordinary advances in the therapy of both benign and malignant surgical diseases of various organ sites. Much of this progress has been evident over the past decade with new concepts and techniques of management that allow the surgeon to integrate this discipline with medicine, pharmacology, immunology, biostatistics, pathology, genetics, medical and radiation oncology, and diagnostic radiology and imaging. Further, each of these major disciplines contributes a small component for the diagnostic and therapeutic approaches to clinical care; hence the comprehensive planning, integration, and provision of patient care throughout the preoperative, intraoperative, and postoperative phases of care remains essential in the successful practice of our specialty.

The editors acknowledge that the aim of this work is to provide an illustrative, instructive, and comprehensive review that depicts the rationale of basic operative principles essential to surgical therapy. In organizing this monograph, the editors chose authors renowned in the disciplines for illustrating, forming, and depicting in a comprehensive fashion the surgical therapy expectant for metabolic, infectious, endocrine, and neoplastic abnormalities in adult and pediatric patients **from a truly international and multi-continental perspective.** The editors and authors were chosen carefully from across geographies and also from multi-cultural and diverse locations. While the authors consider this text to be inclusive regarding the technical and operative conditions for perioperative care in this field, its purpose should not be intended to replace standard textbooks of surgery nor should it be considered complete in its coverage of pathophysiologic disorders. In contrast, this monograph is organized to familiarize practicing surgeons, residents, and fellows with state-of-the-art surgical principles and techniques essential to contemporary practice. Therefore, the tenor of this monograph on liver and biliary surgery has been developed to coexist with other major surgical reference texts that are dedicated—some in more comprehensive fashion—to the therapy of individual organs of systemic diseases. This monograph is much more a "working text" for the practicing surgeon with emphasis on diagnosis and treatment of liver and biliary disorders. Along with this monograph, nine other paperback monographs are available and focus on the general principles of surgery, trauma, critical care, esophagus and stomach, small bowel, colorectal, pancreas and spleen, oncology, and endocrine organs, all adapted from the primary textbook—*General Surgery: International Principles and Practice.*

The chapters in this monograph on liver and biliary surgery include a condensed bibliography of highly selective journal articles, reviews, and text. In this manner of attempting to be concise, we hope to provide a precise focus for the education of the reader relative to accepted surgical principles involved in patient care. Moreover, the editors have sought to provide a counterpoint view for the selection of therapy by presenting at the opening of each chapter a list of "Pearls and Pitfalls" that highlight particular concerns or controversies. The chapters provide pertinent, though not exhaustive, summaries of anatomy and physiology, a history of surgical illness, and stages of operative approaches with relevant technical considerations outlined in an easily under-standable manner. Complications are reviewed when appropriate for the organ system, diseases, and problem. The text is supported amply by line drawings and photographs that depict anatomic or technical principles. The editors have made every attempt to minimize duplicative or repetitive discussions except when controversial or state-of-the-art issues are presented. Moreover, the editors have attempted to ensure that accurate presentations and illustrations depict properly the most complex problems confronted by the general surgeon.

Finally, in an attempt to address advances in contemporary concepts, the text has been organized to address in detail expeditious, safe, and anatomically accurate operations and incorporate standard as well as evolving surgical principles and techniques. These principles have been tested in the clinics of valid scientific knowledge and are well supported by the time-tested approaches that have been provided by practicing surgeons. The editors are excited to be able to respond to the challenge of developing a truly international text and are indeed hopeful that our readers will find this focused monograph on liver and biliary surgery to be a repository of insight, useful, and timely information.

Kirby I. Bland
Michael G. Sarr
Markus W. Büchler
Attila Csendes
O. James Garden
John Wong

Contents

Part I   Liver—Benign

1   **Hepatitis**..   3
    John J. Poterucha

2   **Differential Diagnosis of the Liver Mass**....................   25
    Wei-Chen Lee and Miin-Fu Chen

3   **Benign Hepatic Neoplasms**   37
    Juan Hepp

4   **Hepatic Abscess: Current Concepts**   53
    Sanchez M. William and Hernando O. Abaunza

5   **Portal Hypertension**   69
    Héctor Orozco and Miguel Angel Mercado

6   **Cystic Liver Diseases**.......................................   85
    Catherine Hubert, Laurence Annet,
    Bernard E.VanBeers, Yves Horsmans,
    and Jean-Franççois Gigot

7   **Liver Transplantation for Budd-Chiari**
    Syndrome..   111
    François Durand and Jacques Belghiti

8 Liver Hemangioma... 125
  Alexis Laurent, Alain Luciani, and Daniel Cherqui

Part II Liver—Malignant

9 Hepatocellular Carcinoma 137
  Sheung Tat Fan

10 Metastatic Cancer of the Liver.................................... 157
  Matteo Donadon, Gareth Morris-Stiff,
  and Jean-Nicolas Vauthey

Part III Biliary Benign

11 Postcholecystectomy Syndrome.................................. 181
  Frank G. Moody

12 Asymptomatic Gallstones.. 191
  Robert V. Rege

13 Bile Duct Injury Following Laparoscopic
  Cholecystectomy 201
  Stephen A. Boyce and O. James Garden

14 Cholelithiasis.. 221
  Luis A. Ibañez, Jean M. Butte, and Nicolás A. Devaud

15 Choledocholithiasis 235
  Toshiyuki Mori, Yutaka Suzuki,
  Masanori Sugiyama, and Yutaka Atomi

16 Choledochal Cysts 257
  Chi-Leung Liu

17 Biliary Dyskinesia: Functional Gallbladder
  and Sphincter of Oddi Disorders.................................. 265
  Cary B. Aarons, Arthur F. Stucchi,
  and James M. Becker

18 Primary Sclerosing Cholangitis.................................... 289
Nicholas J. Zyromski and Henry A. Pitt

Part IV   Biliary—Malignant

19 Perihilar Cholangiocarcinoma 307
Yuji Nimura and Hideki Nishio

20 Cancer of the Gallbladder.. 317
Xabier A. de Aretxabala and Ivan S. Roa

Part V   Minimally Invasive Procedures

21 Laparoscopic Common Bile Duct Exploration 335
Leslie Karl Nathanson

Index... 349

Contributors

Cary B. Aarons, MD
General Surgery Resident, Department of Surgery, Boston University Medical Center, Boston, MA, USA

Hernando Abaunza O., MD, FACS
Professor, Department of Surgery, Universidad Nacional de Colombia, Hospital Militar Central, Bogota, Colombia

Laurence Annet, MD, PhD
Department of Radiology, Saint-Luc University Hospital, Université Catholique de Louvain, Brussels, Belgium

Yutaka Atomi, MD, PhD, FACS
Professor of Surgery, Department of Surgery, School of Medicine, Kyorin University, Tokyo, Japan

James M. Becker, MD, FACS
James Utley Professor and Chairman, Department of Surgery, Boston University Medical Center, Boston, MA, USA

Jacques Belghiti, MD
Professor, Department of Digestive Surgery, Hospital Beaujon, Clichy, France

Stephen A. Boyce, BA, MBBS, MRCS
Specialist Registrar, Department of Surgery, University of Edinburgh Royal Infirmary of Edinburgh, Edinburgh, UK

Jean M. Butte, MD
Faculty of Medicine, Department of Digestive Surgery,
Pontificia Universidad Católica de Chile, Santiago, Chile

Miin-Fu Chen, MD, FACS
Professor and Director, Department of General Surgery,
Chang-Gung Memorial Hospital, Chang-Gung University,
Taoyuan, Taiwan, Republic of China

Daniel Cherqui, MD
Professor and Chief, Department of Digestive Surgery,
CHU Henri Mondor, Creteil, France

Xabier A. de Aretxabala, MD, FACS
Professor, Department of Surgery, Clinic Hospital
University of Chile, Santiago, Chile

Nicolás A. Devaud, MD
Department of Digestive Surgery, Pontificia Universidad
Católica de Chile, Santiago, Chile

Matteo Donadon, MD
Clinical Research Fellow, Department of Surgical Oncology,
The University of Texas M D Anderson Cancer Center,
Houston, TX, USA

François Durand, MD
Staff Surgeon, Department of Hepatology, Hospital
Beaujon, Clichy, France

Sheung Tat Fan, MBBS, MS, MD, PhD, DSc, FRCS, FACS, FCSHK, FHKAM
Professor and Chairman of Hepatobiliary Surgery, Head,
Department of Surgery, University of Hong Kong, Queen
Mary Hospital, Hong Kong, China

O. James Garden, MBChB, MD, FRCS(Ed), FRCP(Ed), FRACS(Hon)
Regius Professor of Clinical Surgery, Department of Clinical and Surgical Sciences, The University of Edinburgh, Royal Infirmary of Edinburgh, Edinburgh, UK

Jean-François Gigot, MD, PhD, FRCS
Professor, Surgical Hepatobiliary and Pancreatic Division, Saint-Luc University Hospital, Brussels, Belgium

Juan Hepp, MC
Department of Surgery, Clínica Alemana, Santiago, Santiago, Chile

Catherine Hubert, MD
Surgical Hepatobiliary and Pancreatic Division, Saint-Luc University Hospital, Université Catholique de Louvain (UCL), Brussels, Belgium

Yves Horsmans, MD, PhD
Professor, Department of Gastro-Enterology, Saint-Luc University Hospital, Université Catholique de Louvain (UCL), Brussels, Belgium

Luis A. Ibañez, MD
Professor of Surgery and Head, Department of Digestive Surgery, Pontificia Universidad Católica de Chile, Santiago, Chile

Alexis Laurent, MD, PhD
Department of Digestive Surgery, CHU Henri Mondor, Créteil, France

Wei-Chen Lee, MD
Department of Liver Surgery and Transplantation, Chang-Gung Memorial Hospital, Chang-Gung University, Taoyuan, Taiwan, Republic of China

Chi-Leung Liu, MBBS, MS, MD, FRCS, FACS
Associate Professor, Department of Surgery, University
of Hong Kong, Queen Mary Hospital, Hong Kong, China

Alain Luciani, MD
Department of Imagerie Medicale, CHU Henri Mondor,
Creteil, France

Miguel Angel Mercado, MD
Professor and Chief, Department of Surgery, Instituto
Nacional de Ciencias, Medicasy Nutricion, Mexico City,
Mexico

Frank G. Moody, MD
Professor, Department of Surgery, University of Texas
Medical School, Houston, TX, USA

Toshiyuki Mori, MD, FACS
Associate Professor, Department of Surgery, School
of Medicine, Kyorin University, Tokyo, Japan

Gareth J. Morris-Stiff, MBBCh, MD, MCh, FRCS
Specialist, Registrar, Department of Laparoscopic Surgery,
Princess of Wales, Hospital Bridgend, UK

Leslie Karl Nathanson, MBChB, FRACS
Department of Surgery, Royal Brisbane Hospital, Brisbane,
Australia

Yuji Nimura, MD
President, Aichi Cancer Center Hospital and Research
Institute, Nagoya, Japan

Hideki Nishio, MD
Lecturer, Department of Surgery, Nagoya University
Graduate School of Medicine, Nagoya, Japan

Héctor Orozco, MD FACS
Professor and Chairman, Surgical Division, Instituto
Nacional de Ciencias Medicas y Nutricion, Mexico City,
Mexico

Henry A. Pitt, MD
Professor, Department of Surgery, Indiana University,
Indianapolis, IN, USA

John J. Poterucha, MD
Associate Professor of Medicine, Division of
Gastroenterology and Hepatology, Mayo Clinic College
of Medicine, Rochester, MN, USA

Robert V. Rege, MD
Professor and Chairman, Department of Surgery, The
University of Texas Southwestern Medical Center at Dallas,
Dallas, TX, USA

Ivan S. Roa, MD
Chief, Department of Pathology, Clinica Alemana Santiago,
Universidad de la Frontera, Santiago, Chile

William Sanchez M., MD, FACS
Associate Professor of Surgery, Universidad Militar Nueva
Granada, Hospital Militar Central, Bogota, Colombia

Arthur F. Stucchi, PhD
Associate Research Professor Department of Surgery,
Pathology and Laboratory Medicine Boston University
School of Medicine Boston, MA, USA

Masanori Sugiyama, MD, PhD
Professor, Department of Surgery, School of Medicine,
Kyorin University, Tokyo, Japan

Yutaka Suzuki, MD, PhD
Department of Surgery, School of Medicine, Kyorin
University, Tokyo, Japan

Bernard E. Van Beers, MD, PhD
Professor of Radiology, Department of Medical Imaging,
Saint-Luc University Hospital, Université Catholique de
Louvain (UCL), Brussels, Belgium

Jean-Nicholas Vauthey, MD, FACS
Professor of Surgery, Department of Surgical Oncology,
University of Texas M D Anderson Cancer Center, Houston,
TX, USA

Nicholas J. Zyromski, MD
Assistant Professor of Surgery, Department of Surgery,
Indiana University, Indianapolis, IN, USA

Part I
Liver—Benign

1
Hepatitis

John J. Poterucha

Pearls and Pitfalls

- Increases in serum aminotransferases are indicative of hepatocellular injury, while increases in alkaline phosphatase suggest biliary injury, inflammation, or obstruction.
- Increases in serum bilirubin concentration can be secondary to intrahepatic cholestasis (hepatocellular pathology) or mechanical biliary obstruction.
- The best judge of hepatic function may be the prothrombin time (INR).
- Non-alcoholic fatty liver disease (NAFLD) is becoming a major cause of liver disease and cirrhosis.
- The most common causes of viral hepatitis are hepatitis A, B, and C.
- Hepatitis A infection is self-limited without chronic disease.
- Hepatitis B is transmitted by needle stick or sexual contact. Hepatitis B accounts for 40% of acute viral hepatitis and 15% of chronic viral hepatitis.
- Diagnosis of hepatitis B infection is made by hepatitis B surface antigen (HBs Ag).
- All healthcare workers should be immunized against HBV infection.

K.I. Bland et al. (eds.), *Liver and Biliary Surgery*,
DOI 10.1007/978-1-84996-429-6_1,
© Springer-Verlag London Limited 2011

- Hepatitis C causes 20% of acute viral hepatitis, 60% of chronic hepatitis, and about 40% of all end-stage liver disease in the USA.
- Diagnosis of hepatitis C involves anti-hepatitis C viral antibodies (anti-HCV) or hepatitis C viral RNA (HCV-RNA).
- Sixty percent to 85% of persons with HCV infection remain chronically infected, of whom 20% will develop cirrhosis.

Introduction

There are many causes of liver injury and knowledge of the more common disorders is important to the surgeon. Hepatitis viruses are common causes of liver injury and their clinical importance should be recognized, not only because of their propensity for liver injury, but also because of the risk of transmission. The purpose of this chapter is to familiarize the surgeon with a practical approach to patients with liver disease with an emphasis on the agents that result in viral hepatitis. This chapter will be divided into four major sections:

A. Evaluation of the patient with abnormal liver tests
B. Viral hepatitis
C. Post-operative liver injury
D. Risk of surgery in patients with liver disease

Evaluation of the Patient with Abnormal Liver Tests

The evaluation of patients with abnormal liver blood tests hinges on many clinical factors including the patient's symptoms, age, risk factors for liver disease, personal or family history of liver disease, medications, and findings on physical examination. Because of these multiple factors, designing a standard algorithm for the evaluation of liver test abnormalities is difficult. It is important to understand the commonly used liver tests, the differential diagnosis of diseases characterized by increases in aminotransferases versus alkaline phosphatase, and evaluation of the jaundiced patient.

Commonly Used Liver Tests

Aminotransferases (ALT, AST): Aminotransferases (also referred to as transaminases) are enzymes located in the cytoplasm of hepatocytes and are therefore markers of hepatocellular disease. Injury to hepatocyte membrane allows these enzymes to "leak" out of liver cells, resulting in increases in serum within a few hours after liver injury. Aminotransferases consist of the alanine aminotransferase (ALT), also known in the past as serum glutamate pyruvate transaminase (SGPT) and aspartate aminotransferase (AST), or serum glutamate oxaloacetate transaminase (SGOT). ALT is more specific for liver injury than AST.

Alkaline phosphatase: In contrast, alkaline phosphatase is an enzyme in the hepatocyte membrane bordering bile canaliculi and is more representative of bile duct obstruction or inflammation rather than hepatocyte injury. Because alkaline phosphatase is also found in bone and placenta, an isolated increase in the enzyme should prompt further testing to see if the origin is from liver or other tissues; determination of alkaline phosphatase *isoenzymes* is one such way. Another marker of liver injury is serum gamma-glutamyltransferase (GGT), an enzyme of intrahepatic biliary canaliculi. Other than to confirm the hepatic origin of an increased alkaline phosphatase, GGT has little role in the determination of diseases of the liver, because its synthesis can be induced by many medications thus reducing its specificity for *clinically significant* liver disease. Alkaline phosphatase has to be upregulated and synthesized before it is released, and therefore, diseases characterized by acute biliary obstruction, such as might occur with a common bile duct stone, may not result initially in an increase in alkaline phosphatase.

Bilirubin: Serum bilirubin is measured in direct (conjugated) and indirect (unconjugated) fractions. Commonly occurring liver diseases generally lead to an increase in both direct and indirect fractions. Hepatocyte dysfunction or impairment of bile flow will cause hyperbilirubinemia that is usually ≥50% conjugated. Diseases characterized by overproduction of bilirubin, such as hemolysis or resorption of a hematoma, are characterized by hyperbilirubinemia that is ≤20% conjugated.

Prothrombin time and albumin: Prothrombin time (measured as international normalized ratio, INR) and serum albumin are markers of the synthetic function of the liver and are probably the best overall markers of severity of liver disease. Abnormalities in INR and albumin imply severe liver disease and should prompt immediate evaluation. Hepatocellular dysfunction is characterized by an inability to synthesize clotting factors despite adequate stores of vitamin K. A prolonged INR due to vitamin K deficiency may be produced by antibiotics associated with a prolonged period of fasting, malabsorptive disorders such as celiac disease, or severe cholestasis with an inability to absorb fat-soluble vitamins (e.g. vitamin K). Correction of the INR after administration of vitamin K documents vitamin K deficiency rather than impaired hepatocellular function.

Because serum albumin has a half-life of 21 days, decreases due to liver dysfunction are not apparent acutely; however, serum albumin can decrease relatively quickly in a patient with severe systemic illness such as bacteremia. These rapid decreases are likely secondary to cytokine release with accelerated metabolism of albumin. A decrease of albumin in a patient without overt liver disease should prompt consideration of albumin loss in the urine or gastrointestinal tract.

Hepatocellular Disorders

Diseases affecting primarily hepatocytes are said to cause "hepatitis" and are characterized by predominant increases in serum aminotransferases with normal or lesser increases in serum alkaline phosphatase. Hepatitis generally is subdivided based on disease duration into acute or chronic (duration arbitrarily defined as less than or greater than 3 months). Patients with acute hepatitis often have fatigue, nausea, mild upper abdominal pain, and jaundice; aminotransferases are usually >500 U/L (normal values are <40–45 U/L). The abdominal pain of acute hepatitis is usually less severe than that of biliary duct obstruction. Increased liver tests or jaundice without a clear history of biliary pain is not an indication for cholecystectomy. The more common causes of acute hepatitis are listed in Table 1.1.

The degree and pattern of increases in aminotransferases may be helpful in the differential diagnosis of acute hepatitis. Acute hepatitis due to *viruses or drugs other than acetaminophen* generally produces increases in aminotransferase of 1,000–3,000 U/L. In general, ALT is greater than AST. ALT >5,000 U/L is usually due to acetaminophen hepatotoxicity, hepatic ischemia ("shock liver"), or an unusual virus such as herpes. The *hepatic ischemia* that occurs after an episode of hypotension, usually in patients with pre-existing cardiac disease, leads to very high serum aminotransferases that

TABLE 1.1. Common causes of acute hepatitis.

Disease	Clinical clues	Diagnostic tests
Hepatitis A	Exposure history	IgM anti-HAV
Hepatitis B	Risk factors	HBsAg, IgM anti-HBc
Drug-induced	Compatible medication/timing	Improvement after withdrawal from agent
Alcoholic hepatitis	History of alcohol excess, AST:ALT > 2	Liver biopsy, improvement with abstinence
Ischemic hepatitis	History of hypotension	Rapid improvement of aminotransferases
Acute duct obstruction	Abdominal pain, fever	Cholangiogram

See text for abbreviations.

improve dramatically within a few days. Another cause of a short-lived increase in aminotransferases is transient bile duct obstruction, usually due to a stone. These increases can be as high as 1,000 U/L but improve within 24–48 h. Patients with transient bile duct obstruction usually have prominent abdominal pain. *Alcoholic hepatitis* is characterized by more modest increases in aminotransferase, always less than 400 IU and at times near normal. Patients with alcoholic hepatitis also usually have an AST:ALT ratio greater than 2 and frequently have an increases serum bilirubin out of proportion to the aminotransferase elevations.

Diseases producing sustained (>3–6 months) increases in aminotransferases are said to be causing chronic hepatitis. In general, these increases in aminotransferase are more modest than those in acute hepatitis, usually 2–5 fold increased. Most patients with chronic hepatitis are asymptomatic, although some patients have fatigue and mild right upper quadrant pain. The differential diagnosis of chronic hepatitis is relatively lengthy, but the most important and common disorders are found in Table 1.2.

Risk factors for *hepatitis C* include a history of blood transfusions or intravenous drug use. Patients with *hepatitis B*

TABLE 1.2. Common causes of chronic hepatitis.

Disease	Clinical clues	Diagnostic tests
Hepatitis C	Risk factors	Anti-HCV
Hepatitis B	Risk factors	HBsAg
Nonalcoholic steatohepatitis	Obesity, diabetes, hyperlipidemia	Ultrasonography, liver biopsy
Hemochromatosis	Arthritis, diabetes, family history	Iron studies, gene test, biopsy
Alcoholic liver disease	History, AST:ALT > 2	Liver biopsy
Autoimmune hepatitis	ALT 200–1,500, usually female, other autoimmune disease	Antinuclear or anti-smooth muscle antibody, biopsy

See text for abbreviations.

may give a history of illegal drug use or frequent sexual contacts or be from a high endemic area such as Asia or Africa. *Nonalcoholic fatty liver disease (NAFLD)* is probably the most common cause of abnormal liver enzymes in the US. Patients with NAFLD usually have obesity, diabetes, and/or hyperlipidemia. Ultrasonography may show changes in echotexture of the liver consistent with fatty infiltration. A careful history will be necessary to help diagnose *drug-induced* or *alcohol-induced* liver disease. Most patients with *genetic hemochromatosis* have normal liver enzymes unless cirrhosis is present, although all will have excess hepatic iron deposition. Genetic hemochromatosis also causes diabetes, hypogonadism, and joint complaints. *Autoimmune hepatitis* may present as an acute or chronic hepatitis; patients usually have aminotransferases of 300–2,000 U/L, a bit greater than other chronic hepatidities. The presence of autoantibodies, hypergammaglobulinemia, and other autoimmune disorders are helpful clues to the diagnosis of autoimmune hepatitis. Low level positive antinuclear antibodies are very common in other forms of chronic liver disease and are therefore not pathognomonic of autoimmune hepatitis.

Cholestatic Disorders

Diseases that affect predominantly the biliary system are termed cholestatic diseases. These processes can affect the microscopic ducts (e.g. primary biliary cirrhosis), large bile ducts (e.g. pancreatic cancer causing common bile duct obstruction), or both (e.g. primary sclerosing cholangitis). In general, the predominant biochemical abnormality in these disorders is in alkaline phosphatase. Although diseases that produce elevations in bilirubin are often called "cholestatic," severe hepatocellular injury, such as occurs with an acute hepatitis, will also produce hyperbilirubinemia because of hepatocellular dysfunction. Common causes of cholestasis are illustrated in Table 1.3.

TABLE 1.3. Common causes of cholestasis.

Disease	Clinical clues	Diagnostic tests
Primary biliary cirrhosis	Middle-aged female	Antimitochondrial antibody
Primary sclerosing cholangitis	Association with ulcerative colitis	Cholangiography (ERCP)
Large bile duct obstruction	Jaundice and pain	Ultrasonography, ERCP
Drug-induced	Compatible medication/timing	Improvement after withdrawal of agent
Intrahepatic mass lesions	History of malignancy	Ultrasonography, computed tomography
Infiltrative disorder	Features of sarcoid or amyloid	Biopsy

Large bile duct obstruction is often due to stones or benign or malignant strictures. Remember that acute large duct obstruction from a stone may produce early on, marked increases in aminotransferases, usually in the setting of biliary-type pain. Most patients with large duct obstruction will have dilated ducts on cross-sectional imaging such as ultrasonography, computed tomography, or magnetic resonance imaging. *Primary sclerosing cholangitis (PSC)* has a strong association with ulcerative colitis. Patients with PSC and PBC are often asymptomatic but may have jaundice, fatigue, or pruritus. *Primary biliary cirrhosis* (PBC) most commonly affects middle-aged women. *Intrahepatic mass lesions* should be considered in a patent with cholestatic liver test abnormalities and a history of malignancy. Any systemic inflammatory process such as infection or immune disorder may produce nonspecific abnormalities in liver tests, usually manifest by a mixed cholestatic (alkaline phosphatase) and hepatocellular (ALT or AST) pattern. NAFLD occasionally produces an increased alkaline phosphatase, while patients with alcoholic hepatitis commonly have an increased alkaline phosphatase.

Jaundice

Jaundice becomes evident visibly when serum bilirubin is >2.5 mg/dl. As noted above, it may be important to note whether the serum bilirubin is predominantly conjugated or unconjugated. A common benign disorder that produces an unconjugated hyperbilirubinemia (although not usually jaundice) is *Gilbert's syndrome*, which affects ~2% of the population. The total bilirubin is generally less than 3.0 mg/dl, while the direct will be 0.3 mg/dl or less. The bilirubin is generally greater in the fasting state or when the patient is ill. A presumptive diagnosis of Gilbert's disease can be made in an otherwise well patient with unconjugated hyperbilirubinemia, normal liver enzymes, and normal hemoglobin (to exclude hemolysis).

Patients with jaundice due to liver or biliary disorders have direct hyperbilirubinemia. The first goal is to differentiate intrahepatic diseases, such as alcoholic or viral hepatitis, from those with obstruction. Abdominal pain, fever, and/or a palpable gallbladder are suggestive of obstruction. Excess intake of alcohol, risk factors for viral hepatitis, a bilirubin greater than 15 mg/dl, and persistent markedly increased aminotransferases suggest that the jaundice is due to hepatocellular dysfunction. In patients with acute hepatocellular dysfunction and jaundice, improvement in bilirubin often lags behind improvement in serum aminotransferase. Computed tomography and ultrasonography are good initial tests to assess for obstructive causes of jaundice. Diseases characterized by large duct obstruction will generally exhibit intrahepatic bile duct dilatation. A common error is to attribute jaundice to extrahepatic bile duct obstruction or gallstones. Operations in patients with intrahepatic cholestasis are complicated commonly by worsening liver function, including life-threatening complications of portal hypertension. Sepsis can also produce jaundice by causing intrahepatic cholestasis.

Viral Hepatitis

Viral hepatitis is important both to surgeons and surgical patients, not only because hepatitis viruses result in clinically relevant liver disease, but also because of the risk of transmission. Viral infections are important causes of liver disease worldwide with five primary hepatitis viruses having been identified (hepatitis A, B, C, D, and E).

Disorders that cause hepatitis are characterized primarily by increases in aminotransferase (ALT and AST). Causes of hepatitis other than viruses include medications, nonalcoholic or alcoholic steatohepatitis, autoimmune hepatitis, or Wilson's disease. Non-hepatotropic viruses, such as cytomegalovirus or Epstein-Barr virus, can also result in hepatitis as part of a systemic infection.

It is useful to divide hepatitis syndromes into acute or chronic. Acute hepatitis can last from weeks up to 3–6 months and is often accompanied by jaundice. The symptoms of acute hepatitis are similar regardless of etiology and include anorexia, malaise, dark urine, fever, and occasionally abdominal pain. The abdominal pain accompanying hepatitis is located generally in the right upper quadrant of the abdomen, is usually mild and constant, and should not be confused with the more severe episodic pain associated with disorders of the biliary tract and pancreas. Chronic hepatitis is defined as the presence of hepatitis for more than 3–6 months. Patients with chronic hepatitis are often asymptomatic but may complain of fatigue. Occasionally, patients have manifestations of cirrhosis (ascites, variceal bleeding, or encephalopathy) as the initial symptoms of a chronic liver disorder. Each primary hepatitis virus causes acute hepatitis, but only hepatitis viruses B, C, and D result in chronic hepatitis (Table 1.4).

Hepatitis A

Hepatitis A virus (HAV) causes about 30% of acute hepatitis in the US Acquisition of hepatitis A requires exposure to contaminated food or infected individuals. Groups at particularly

TABLE 1.4. Comparison of the primary hepatitis viruses.

	HAV	HBV	HDV	HCV	HEV
Incubation (days)	15–50	30–160	Unknown	14–160	14–45
Jaundice	Common	Common	Common	Uncommon	Common
Course	Acute	Acute or chronic	Acute or chronic	Acute or chronic	Acute
Transmission	Fecal-oral	Parenteral	Parenteral	Parenteral	Fecal-oral
Test for diagnosis	IgM Anti-HAV	HBsAg	Anti-HDV	Anti-HCV or HCV-RNA	Anti-HEV

See text for abbreviations.

high risk for acquiring hepatitis A include people living in or traveling to underdeveloped countries, children in day-care centers, homosexual men, and perhaps individuals ingesting raw shellfish. The incubation period for hepatitis A is 2–6 weeks.

The most important determinant of the severity of acute hepatitis A is the age at which infection occurs. Those infected when less than 6 years of age are often asymptomatic and if symptoms are present, rarely include jaundice. Up to 40% of individuals over 40 years of age have serologic evidence of a remote hepatitis A infection, yet neither the patient nor a parent will recall an episode of jaundice. Adults acquiring hepatitis A are much more likely than young children to have jaundice.

Diagnosis of acute hepatitis A is made by the presence of IgM anti-HAV which appears at the onset of the acute phase of the illness and disappears in 3–6 months. IgG anti-HAV also becomes positive during the acute phase and persists for decades. A patient with IgG anti-HAV, but not IgM anti-HAV, has had an infection in the remote past or has received hepatitis A vaccine.

Hepatitis A is almost always a self-limited infection, although there may be a prolonged cholestatic phase characterized by persistence of jaundice for 1–3 months. Rarely, acute hepatitis A may cause fulminant hepatic failure and require liver transplantation. Hepatitis A does not result in chronic infection and should not be in the differential diagnosis of a chronic hepatitis.

Treatment of hepatitis A is supportive. Isolation of hospitalized patients is recommended, although viral titers are actually highest in the presymptomatic phase. Immune globulin should be administered to all household and intimate (including day-care) contacts within 2 weeks of exposure. Hepatitis A vaccine is recommended for individuals with contact to patients with hepatitis A, those planning prolonged stays in areas where hepatitis A is endemic, and persons with chronic liver disease.

Because HAV does not cause chronic infection, parenteral transmission (including that from needle-stick exposure) is rare. Hepatitis A, like any acute hepatitis, may result in jaundice, and the surgeon needs to differentiate the jaundice associated with acute hepatitis from that due to obstruction (see above).

Hepatitis B

Hepatitis B virus (HBV) is a DNA virus that causes about 40% of acute viral hepatitis and 15% of chronic viral hepatitis in the US. Most infected people living currently in the US are immigrants from countries in Asia and Africa with a high prevalence of hepatitis B who likely acquired hepatitis B perinatally or in early childhood. HBV may also be transmitted by needlestick exposure or sexual contact.

The incubation period after HBV infection ranges from 30 to 180 days. Clinical outcome varies. Acute hepatitis B in the adolescent or adult is icteric in 30%. Most patients recover after an episode of acute hepatitis B, although about 5% of infected adults will have persistence of HBsAg (see Table 1.5 for a guide to hepatitis B serologic markers) for longer than 6 months and are termed chronically infected. The outcome of chronic infection is also variable. Some patients have normal liver enzymes, HBV DNA level < 20,000 U/ml, and a normal liver biopsy despite the persistence of HBsAg. Such patients are

TABLE 1.5. Hepatitis B: serological markers.

Test	Significance
HBsAg	Marker for current infection
anti-HBs	Marker for immunity (resolved infection or immunization)
IgM anti-HBc	Suggests recent infection
IgG anti-HBc	Marker for remote infection
HBeAg and HBV-DNA level > 20,000 IU/ml	Marker for active viral replication (high infectivity)

HBsAg = hepatitis B surface antigen; Anti-HBs = antibody to hepatitis B surface; anti-HBc = antibody to hepatitis B core; HBeAg = hepatitis B e antigen; HBV-DNA = hepatitis B virus DNA.

termed HBV inactive carriers and have an excellent prognosis. Individuals with abnormal liver tests and an HBV DNA level > 20,000 U/ml in the setting of chronic HBsAg positivity have chronic hepatitis B and are at much higher risk for developing cirrhosis and hepatocellular carcinoma. Spontaneous clearance of HBsAg occurs in 1–2% of chronically infected patients per year although is even less likely in those who have been infected since early childhood.

Seroconversion of hepatitis B antigen (HBeAg) positive to negative with development of antibody to hepatitis B e (anti-HBe) occurs in about 10% of chronic HBV patients per year and may be accompanied by a flare of disease. Patients with chronic hepatitis B who are HBeAg-negative but have HBV DNA > 20,000 U/ml (HBeAg-negative chronic hepatitis B), are often infected with pre-core or core promoter variants of HBV and may have a worse prognosis than those with wild-type virus.

In general, treatment is given to those patients with hepatitis B who are at risk for progression. Such patients include those with liver enzymes greater than twice the upper limit of normal and active viral replication as defined by HBV-DNA > 20,000 U/ml. Some treatment guidelines also recommend liver biopsy before treatment, especially in patients with only modest abnormalities of liver enzymes. Treatment for hepatitis B can be with pegylated interferon or one of the oral agents, lamivudine, adefovir, entecavir, and telbivudine. Predictors of greater likelihood of response include higher ALT, lower HBV DNA level, shorter duration of disease, and female gender. About 20–30% of patients treated with oral agents have seroconversion of HBeAg after 1–2 years of therapy; treatment should be continued for at least 6 months after seroconversion. Patients without seroconversion of HBeAg need treatment indefinitely. Seroconversion of HBsAg (i.e. cure) with the oral antiviral agents occurs only rarely and should not be considered a reasonable treatment goal.

HBV may be transmitted by needle-stick exposure. Patients with chronic hepatitis B (HBsAg-positive) who have HBV DNA levels > 20,000 IU/ml are at greatest risk for transmitting infection. Health care workers exposed to needles from

HBeAg-positive individuals have a 30% risk of contracting hepatitis B if not already immune. All surgeons should receive the hepatitis B vaccine and verify immunity by measuring anti-HBs 6 months after vaccination and then every 5 years thereafter. Non-immune surgeons exposed to a needle-stick from a HBsAg-positive patient should receive hepatitis B immune globulin as soon as possible after exposure.

Surgeons should also be aware that hepatitis B can still be transmitted rarely by transfusion of blood products. It is estimated that one of every 63,000 units of blood transfused is tainted with hepatitis B. Surgeons may also transmit hepatitis B rarely to patients. Although routine hepatitis B testing of health care workers is not advised, individuals who perform invasive procedures and who do not develop anti-HBs after vaccination should know their HBsAg status, and if positive, the HBeAg and HBV DNA status. HBsAg-positive surgeons should seek counsel from their local medical society and be considered for therapy.

Hepatitis D

Hepatitis D (HDV or the "delta" agent) is a defective virus that requires the presence of HBsAg to cause disease. HDV infection can occur simultaneously with HBV (coinfection) or as a superinfection in persons with established hepatitis B. Hepatitis D is diagnosed by anti-HDV and should be suspected in a patient with acute hepatitis B or an acute exacerbation of chronic hepatitis B. In the US, intravenous drug users are the group of HBV patients at highest risk for acquiring HDV. Because hepatitis D requires the presence of HBsAg to cause disease, the general implications of hepatitis D to the surgeon are similar to those for hepatitis B.

Hepatitis C

Hepatitis C (HCV) is an RNA virus that infects about four million individuals in the US HCV causes 20% of acute hepatitis, 60% of chronic hepatitis, and about 40% of all end-stage liver disease in the US Clinically recognized acute hepatitis C is unusual, and the importance of hepatitis C lies in its propensity to cause chronic infection. Major risk factors for hepatitis C infection are intravenous drug use and blood transfusion prior to 1992.

The incubation period for HCV ranges from 2 to 22 weeks (mean 7 weeks). Most acute hepatitis C is asymptomatic and anicteric. Fully 60–85% of persons with HCV infection fail to clear the virus by 6 months and develop chronic infection. Up to 30% of patients chronically infected with HCV have persistently normal ALT values. Patients with chronic hepatitis C may have nonspecific symptoms such as fatigue and vague abdominal pain. Occasionally, patients present with extrahepatic manifestations such as vasculitis associated with cryoglobulinemia. Once HCV results in cirrhosis, symptoms are more common and include fatigue or complications of end-stage liver disease.

About 20% of patients with chronic hepatitis C develop cirrhosis over a 10–20 year period. A long duration of infection and alcohol abuse are risk factors for the development of cirrhosis. The rate of progression of hepatitis C is slow, with those patients developing cirrhosis generally doing so only after more than 15 years of disease. Patients with cirrhosis due to HCV are at risk for developing hepatocellular carcinoma and should undergo surveillance with ultrasonography every 6–12 months.

A guide to the interpretations of hepatitis C tests is found in Table 1.6. Antibody to HCV (anti-HCV) is not protective and indicates either current or resolved infection. Anti-HCV by enzyme-linked immunoassay (ELISA) is sensitive for HCV infection and is the screening test of choice in most laboratories. The specificity of the ELISA is improved with the addition of the recombinant immunoblot assay (RIBA). A positive RIBA indicates the presence of antibodies to HCV but still could represent a resolved infection. The presence of HCV-RNA by polymerase chain reaction is diagnostic of ongoing HCV infection. HCV-RNA level and genotype can also be obtained if therapy is being considered.

TABLE 1.6. Interpretation of anti-HCV results.

Anti-HCV by EIA	Anti-HCV by RIBA	Interpretation
Positive	Negative	False positive EIA, patient does not have true antibody
Positive	Positive	Patient has antibody[a]
Positive	Indeterminate	Uncertain antibody status

See text for abbreviations.
[a]Remember that anti-HCV does not necessarily indicate current hepatitis C infection.

Therapy for hepatitis C with pegylated interferon and ribavirin for 6–12 months results in a sustained loss of virus response in about 50–60% of patients. Because of the multiple side effects of treatment and the relatively low response rates, treatment is generally recommended if a biopsy demonstrates substantial fibrosis or the patient has genotypes 2 or 3 (which are more likely to respond than genotype 1). Treatment is less likely to be effective or tolerated in patients with decompensated cirrhosis; such patients should be referred for liver transplantation.

Hepatitis C is spread parenterally and rarely can be spread by needle-stick exposure. Prospective studies demonstrate seroconversion rates of 0% to 11% after a needle-stick exposure from a hepatitis C-positive patient. Unfortunately, there is no hepatitis C vaccine available, and post-exposure prophylaxis has not proven beneficial. After exposure to a hepatitis C positive individual, HCV RNA should be determined in 2–4 weeks and anti-HCV in 3–6 months. In the unlikely event that hepatitis C transmission occurs, treatment with pegylated interferon and ribavirin may be offered.

There are case reports of transmission of HCV from surgeon to patients. Nevertheless, transmission is exceedingly rare, and there are currently no practice limitations for health care workers infected with HCV. Surgeons should also be aware that while blood product transfusion was a common cause of hepatitis C prior to 1990, the virus is now spread only rarely by blood transfusion. Estimates are that only one of every 103,000 units of blood transfused would be infected with HCV.

Hepatitis E

Hepatitis E causes large outbreaks of acute hepatitis in underdeveloped countries. Physicians in the United States are unlikely to see a patient with hepatitis E. A rare patient may become infected during foreign travel. Clinically, hepatitis E infection is similar to hepatitis A. Resolution of the hepatitis is the rule, and chronic infection does not occur.

Differentiation of viral hepatidities: Ordering tests for cases of presumed viral hepatitis can be confusing, but Tables 1.7 and 1-8 give a practical guide for testing for patients presenting with acute or chronic hepatitis.

Post-Operative Liver Injury

Mild abnormalities in liver enzymes are common after general anesthesia. Most individuals undergoing abdominal operations will have decreased hepatic blood flow, which may contribute to these mild abnormalities. A more severe acute hepatitis may occur after general anesthesia and is best described after the use of halothane but may also be seen with other inhaled anesthetic agents. Post-operative jaundice may be due to liver injury, although indirect hyperbilirubinemia occurs occasionally due to resorption of a large hematoma. Ischemic hepatitis only occurs after a sustained hypotensive episode and is characterized by marked increases in aminotransferases that improve relatively quickly but can be followed by jaundice.

Operations on Patients with Liver Disease

The alterations in hepatic blood flow that occur with general anesthesia can cause decompensation in patients with more severe forms of liver disease. Although good data about the

TABLE 1.7. Acute hepatitis: practical guide to ordering tests and interpretations.

Interpretation	Tests to order			
	IgM anti-HAV	HBsAg	IgM anti-HBc	anti-HCV
Acute HAV	Positive	Negative	Negative	Negative
Acute HBV	Negative	Positive	Positive	Negative
Acute HBV[a]	Negative	Negative	Positive	Negative
Chronic HBV[b]	Negative	Positive	Negative	Negative
Acute or chronic HCV[c]	Negative	Negative	Negative	Positive
Exclude other causes[c]	Negative	Negative	Negative	Negative

See text for abbreviations.
[a]Occasionally patients with acute HBV will lack HBsAg.
[b]HBsAg without IgM anti-HBc is more suggestive of chronic HBV. Exclude HDV or other non-viral causes of acute hepatitis.
[c]Anti-HCV may not be positive in acute hepatitis C and, when present, may indicate chronic infection so other causes should be excluded.

TABLE 1.8. Chronic hepatitis: practical guide to ordering tests and interpretation.

Interpretation	Tests to order	
	HBsAg	anti-HCV
HBV	Positive	Negative
HCV	Negative	Positive
Exclude other causes	Negative	Negative

See text for abbreviations.

risks of operation in patients with liver disease are lacking, the more severe the liver disease, the more likely that decompensation may occur. The type of operation may also be important, with the highest rates of decompensation occurring after abdominal or thoracic procedures; however, even relatively minor surgery such as umbilical herniorrhaphy in a patient with cirrhosis may result in worsening of liver disease. Patients with acute hepatitis, severe alcoholic hepatitis, and those with cirrhosis with evidence of hepatic compromise are at the highest risk of post-operative liver injury. In general, more severe forms of liver disease can be identified by the presence of laboratory parameters of abnormal liver function (hyperbilirubinemia, prolonged prothrombin time, or hypoalbuminemia), physical examination, or historical evidence of complications of portal hypertension (ascites, portal systemic encephalopathy, splenomegaly, or varices).

For patients with cirrhosis, outcomes after abdominal operations depend on the severity of liver disease as measured by the Child-Pugh score (see Table 1.9). Mortality rates of 10%, 30%, and 82% have been reported with patients with Child-Pugh class A, B, and C, respectively. Even patients with well-compensated cirrhosis are at risk for death after abdominal operations. Decompensation of the liver disease is even more common and consists usually of development or worsening of ascites, encephalopathy, jaundice, or bleeding. Ascites can be a particular problem after abdominal operations, because it can compromise wound healing. If advanced liver disease is noted at operation, stomas should be avoided if at all possible.

Complication rates after operations on patients with cirrhosis are high enough that nonoperative interventions are preferred if at all possible. In those situations where operative intervention is required, careful monitoring of mental status and fluid status in the postoperative period is especially important. Limiting the amount of sodium-containing intravenous fluids after operation will help prevent ascites.

TABLE 1.9. Child-Pugh classification of severity of liver disease.

	1 point	2 points	3 points
Encephalopathy	None	Grade 1 or 2	Grade 3 or 4
Ascites	None	Mild	Moderate or severe
Bilirubin (mg/dl)	<2	2.1–3	>3
Albumin	>3.5	2.8–3.5	<2.8
Prothrombin time (INR)	<1.7	1.7–2.3	>2.3

Class A = 5–6 points, class B = 7–9 points, and class C = 10–15 points.

Selected Readings

Centers for Disease Control and Prevention (1999) Prevention of hepatitis A through active or passive immunization: recommendations of the Advisory Committee on Immunization Practices (ACIP). Morbidity and Mortality Weekly Report 48 (No. RR–12):1–54

Centers for Disease Control (1997) Immunization of health-care workers: recommendations of the advisory committee on immunization practices and the hospital infection control practices advisory committee. Morbidity and Mortality Weekly Report 46 (RR–18):1–42

Centers for Disease Control (1991) Recommendations for preventing transmission of human immunodeficiency virus and hepatitis B virus to patients during exposure-prone invasive procedures. Morbidity and Mortality Weekly Report 40 (RR–08):1–9

Friedman LS (1999) The risk of surgery in patients with liver disease. Hepatol 29:1617–1623

Ganem D, Prince AM (2004) Hepatitis B virus infection – natural history and clinical consequences. NEJM 350:1118–1129

Keeffe EB, Dieterich DT, Han SB, et al. (2004) A treatment algorithm for the management of hepatitis B infection in the United States. Clin Gastroenterol Hepatol 2:87–106

Lok AS, McMahon BJ (2007) AASLD practice guidelines: chronic hepatitis B. Hepatology 45:507–539

Poterucha JJ (2006) Approach the patient with abnormal liver tests and fulminant liver failure. In: Hauser SC (ed) Mayo Clinic Gastroenterology and Hepatology Board Review. Mayo Clinic Scientific Press, Rochester, pp 263–270

Poterucha JJ Chronic viral hepatitis (2006) In: Hauser SC (ed) Mayo Clinic Gastroenterology and Hepatology Board Review. Mayo Clinic Scientific Press, Rochester, pp 271–280

Schreiber GB, Busch MP, Kleinman SH, et al. (1996) The risk of transfusion-transmitted viral infections. NEJM 334:1685–1690

Strader DB, Wright T, Thomas DL, et al. (2004) AASLD guideline: diagnosis, management, and treatment of hepatitis C. Hepatology 39:1147–1171

2

Differential Diagnosis of the Liver Mass

Wei-Chen Lee and Miin-Fu Chen

Pearls and Pitfalls

- Currently, most liver masses are asymptomatic and are identified incidentally during survey for chronic liver diseases or other purposes.
- Many liver masses occur in cirrhotic livers secondary to chronic hepatitis B virus (HBV) and hepatitis C virus (HCV) infections.
- Abdominal ultrasonography is the most convenient imaging modality to screen patients at risk for liver masses and will differentiate cystic from solid tumors.
- Dynamic computed tomography (CT) is recommended to assess the liver tumor and remainder of the abdominal cavity simultaneously.
- CT, magnetic resonance imaging (MRI), and angiography can be valuable and complementary in the evaluation of liver masses.
- Tumor markers, such as α-fetoprotein (AFP), carcinoembryonic antigen (CEA), and carbohydrate antigen 19-9 (CA19-9), may help to narrow the differential diagnosis.
- Positron emission tomography (PET) has not proven useful or cost-effective for differentiating most liver masses.
- Liver biopsy is recommended only when operative intervention is not planned and a correct diagnosis would alter treatment planning.

K.I. Bland et al. (eds.), *Liver and Biliary Surgery*,
DOI 10.1007/978-1-84996-429-6_2,
© Springer-Verlag London Limited 2011

Introduction

Currently, a majority of liver masses are asymptomatic and are diagnosed incidentally or during screening of patients with liver disease. Prior to the advent of ultrasonography, however, symptomatic or palpable large tumors were common. While identification of the presence of a liver mass is important, it is even more important to make a correct diagnosis.

Several benign and malignant liver tumors exist (Table 2.1). The appropriate management of a liver mass necessitates an accurate differential diagnosis. Frequently, the diagnosis requires a thorough clinical history, physical examination, laboratory assessment, and imaging methods.

Diagnostic Tools

Laboratory evaluation: Liver enzymes, alanine aminotransferase (ALT) and aspartate aminotransferase (AST), hepatitis B antigens, antibody to hepatitis C, AFP, and CEA all should be

TABLE 2.1. Classification of the common liver mass.

Benign	Malignant
Hemangioma	Hepatocellular carcinoma
Focal nodular hyperplasia	Cholangiocarcinoma
Hepatocellular adenoma	Metastatic tumor
Simple cyst	Angiosarcoma
Polycystic liver disease	Cystadenocarcinoma
Cystadenoma	Epithelioid hemangioendothelioma
Abscess	
Angiomyolipoma	
Lipoma	
Inflammation pseudotumor	
Regenerative nodule	
Fat sparing	

measured. HBVs and HCVs are both precipitating factors for hepatocellular carcinoma (HCC). In Southeast Asia, about 60% and 30% of patients with HCC are associated with chronic hepatitis B and hepatitis C infections, respectively. Thus, all the patients having liver tumors should have the profiles of virus infection to make a differential diagnosis. When present, AFP is a virtually diagnostic serum marker for HCC; however, only 65% of HCC patients have an increased serum level of AFP. CEA and CA19-9 are important markers of colorectal and other GI tract cancers, and increased values may indicate biliary or metastatic disease.

Liver ultrasonography: Because abdominal ultrasonography is both noninvasive and inexpensive, currently, it is the imaging method used most frequently to screen for liver tumors. Ultrasonography can effectively identify a liver mass of 5 mm and is valuable to differentiate cystic from solid lesions.

Dynamic computed tomography (CT): CT is the most effective tool to diagnose and evaluate liver masses. Neoplasms demonstrate a preference for arterial blood supply. This physiologic fact allows for differentiating characteristics on diagnostic imaging. Dynamic CT is performed at a time sequence when contrast medium is infused to obtain CT imaging in the arterial phase (25–30 s delay), portal phase (70–80 s delay), and delayed phase (10 min delay). Based on the vascular densities during these different phases, liver tumors can often be differentiated from one another.

Magnetic resonance imaging (MRI): MRI, a noninvasive examination, has a superior soft-tissue contrast and topographic accuracy. Contrast agents to be used with MRI have been developed to increase the accuracy of differential diagnosis. Superparamagnetic iron oxides (SPIO) are iron oxide particles that are taken up by the reticuloendothelial system. For liver imaging studies, intravenous infusion of SPIO reduces signal intensity of the liver parenchyma on T2-weighted images and help distinguish benign and malignant tumors.

Angiography: Angiography is an invasive examination that is used rarely, given the accuracy of noninvasive imaging. By analyzing blood supply and vascular pattern, differentiation of liver masses can be made. Furthermore, with the use of angiography combined with CT, smaller tumors can be identified more often.

Liver biopsy: When the entity of the liver masses cannot be determined by imaging studies, liver biopsy may be indicated; however, in patients with a worrisome lesion who are candidates for resection, biopsy is not necessary or recommended. Complications of biopsy such as intraperitoneal bleeding, intra-liver hematoma, bile leak, or malignancy seeding may occur. Therefore, liver biopsy is generally recommended only when operative resection is contraindicated and definite diagnosis is needed for other treatment planning, or when a lesion is not suspicious and a biopsy would prevent an operation.

Differential Diagnosis

Regenerative nodule: Liver cirrhosis results from hepatocellular necrosis, fibrosis, and regeneration. Because regenerative nodules are common in liver cirrhosis, the most important clinical problem is to distinguish a regenerative nodule from a small HCC. On liver ultrasonography, regenerative nodules are small, hypoechoic nodules. On dynamic CT, regenerative nodules do not enhance the arterial phase. On MRI, regenerative nodules are hypointense on both T1-and T2-weighted images. HCCs are typically hyperintense on T2-weighted images.

Fat sparing: Fat sparing is a focal area of normal liver parenchyma which is not occupied by fatty tissue in an otherwise fatty steatotic liver. On liver ultrasonography, the focal area is hypoechoic and, if one is not careful, can be mistaken for a small liver tumor.

Hemangioma: Hemangiomas, single or multiple, are the most common benign neoplasms of the liver. The sizes can range from several millimeters to more than 20 cm. Most hemangiomas are asymptomatic and are identified incidentally or during evaluation of patients with chronic HBV or HCV infection. Ultrasonography will show a hyperechoic mass, but is not always diagnostic. Non-contrast CT shows a hypodense lesion compared with the surrounding normal liver parenchyma; contrast-enhanced CT demonstrates peripheral, nodular enhancement on arterial and portal phases and is virtually diagnostic for hemangioma (Fig. 2.1). For lesions less than 2 cm, CT may not show this typical pattern, and MRI can assist with the definitive diagnosis. On MRI, a hemangioma is typically hypointense on T1-weighted images and hyperintense on T2-weighted images.

Hepatocellular adenoma: Liver adenomas are rare tumors in the liver and occur predominantly in females who have taken contraceptive pills. Clinically, liver adenomas are identified incidentally or during evaluation of upper abdominal pain which can be due to intra-tumor bleeding. Liver ultrasonography demonstrates a well-defined, hyperechoic tumor. Hemorrhage within the neoplasm will result in a hypoechoic or heteroechoic pattern. Dynamic CT shows a hypervascular appearance with only slight peripheral enhancement on arterial phase and isodense or hyperdense on portal phase. On MRI, liver adenomas demonstrate hyperintense signals in

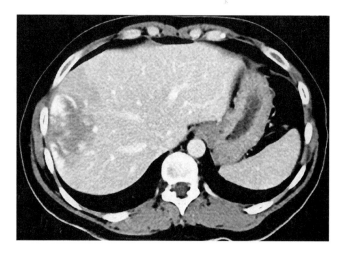

FIGURE 2.1. Dynamic CT of hemangioma. Dynamic CT demonstrates peripheral nodular enhancement on arterial phase.

both T1-and T2-weighted images; however, these imaging appearances are not specific. Liver biopsy may be needed to make a definite diagnosis and avoid the need for resection.

Focal nodular hyperplasia (FNH): FNH is a common benign tumor second in incidence to hemangioma. Liver ultrasonography may demonstrate either a hypoechoic or hyperechoic tumor, which is neither specific nor diagnostic. Dynamic CT will give a hypervascular lesion on arterial phase and isodense or hyperdense lesion on portal phase. Only 30–50% of FNH display the classic central scarring, which will have a linear, hypodense appearance on CT and help to make the diagnosis. On MRI, liver FNH appear hypointense in T1-weighted images and hyperintense in T2-weighted images. If angiography is performed, it usually shows a large central arterial vessel.

Simple cyst and polycystic liver disease: Liver cysts are very common and range from asymptomatic lesions a few millimeters in size to large symptomatic lesions compressing adjacent structures. These cysts are the most common liver abnormality on imaging. Large cysts and polycystic disease may be palpable or cause abdominal pain. Liver ultrasonography or CT is diagnostic and demonstrates round, anechoic lesions with a smooth wall and posterior enhancement.

Abscess: Liver abscesses result from bacteria or parasites. Patients may present with fever and right upper quadrant pain. Ultrasonography demonstrates a round or oval liver lesion, mixed echogenicity on occasion with a fluid/debris level, and an irregular wall. Contrast-enhanced CT typically demonstrates a hypodense lesion with irregular, enhancing walls. Occasionally, gas bubbles or gas-fluid levels can be seen in the cystic lesion.

Angiomyolipoma: Angiomyolipomas are composed of variable amounts of fat, vessels, and muscle, and are seen commonly in the kidney, but only rarely in the liver. Because of the fat content within the mass, liver ultrasonography shows a hyperechoic tumor. On CT, angiomyolipomas are hypodense without contrast enhancement and heterogeneous with contrast enhancement. On MRI, they appear hyperintense on T1-weighted images but more heterointense on the

T2-weighted images. Detection of the fatty component confirms the diagnosis.

Inflammatory pseudotumor: Inflammatory pseudotumors are unusual liver masses, typically identified incidentally. They consist of hepatocytes, fibroblasts, and inflammatory cells. Liver ultrasonography may show either hyperechoic or hypoechoic tumors. On dynamic CT, they appear hyper-vascular on arterial phase and isodense or hyperdense on portal phase. Inflammatory pseudotumors may mimic either benign or malignant neoplasms. Therefore, the differential diagnosis is arduous based on imaging studies alone, and liver biopsy may be necessary to make a definite diagnosis and avoid unnecessary hepatectomy.

Cystadenoma and cystadenocarcinoma: Cystadenomas and cystadenocarcinomas are rare cystic neoplasms in the liver originating from biliary epithelium. Liver ultrasonography demonstrates typically an anechoic cystic lesion with septa-tions or papillary growths from the wall of the cystic area. CT may also demonstrate cystic lesion with septa or papillary growing. Cystadenomas and cystadenocarcinomas cannot be differentiated by imaging studies alone, and surgical resec-tion is usually indicated.

Hepatocellular carcinoma (HCC): HCCs, single or multiple, are the most common primary malignancy in the liver. More than 60% of HCC occurs in cirrhotic livers highly associated with chronic hepatitis B and hepatitis C infections. The defini-tive diagnosis is assisted by laboratory assessment and imag-ing. A serum level of AFP >400 mg/ml in the setting of a suspicious lesion on imaging is virtually pathognomonic of HCC. When the serum level of AFP is <400 mg/ml, but two separate imaging modalities are highly worrisome, HCC is also assumed. Sonographic images of HCC are varied and depend on the size of the neoplasm(s). Small HCCs (<3 cm) are typi-cally hypoechoic, whereas large HCCs are hyperechoic or heteroechoic. The lesions may also have a hypoechoic halo. On dynamic CT, HCCs are hypervascular on the arterial phase and hypodense on the portal phase (Fig. 2.2). On unenhanced MRI or MRI enhanced with SPIO, HCCs are hypointense on

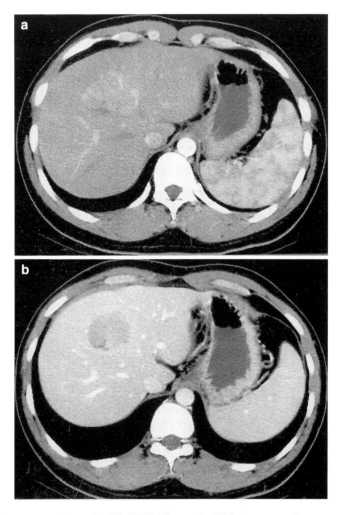

FIGURE 2.2. Dynamic CT of HCC. Dynamic CT demonstrates hypervascular tumors on arterial phase (**a**) and hypodense on portal phase (**b**).

the T1-weighted images but heterointense on the T2-weighted images. However, a mosaic pattern is common for HCC.

Cholangiocarcinoma (CCC): CCC can be divided into central and peripheral types. Central types of CCCs are located most commonly at the liver hilum and cause obstructive jaundice and dilated intrahepatic bile ducts. In contrast, the peripheral types of CCC must be differentiated from other liver tumors. On ultrasonography, the lesion may be hypoechoic, isoechoic, or hyperechoic. On contrast-enhanced CT, peripheral CCCs are ill-defined and nonspecific. On MRI, they appear hypointense in T1-weighted images and hyperintense in T2-weighted images. All the findings of imaging studies, however, are nonspecific and nondiagnostic for peripheral CCCs. Liver biopsy may be needed to make a definite diagnosis.

Metastatic tumor: Metastatic tumors represent the most common malignant neoplasms in the liver. The colon, pancreas, stomach, and breast are the most common primary sites from which these hematogenous metastases arise. Metastatic tumors should be suspected when there are multiple liver tumors or when there is a history of a previous cancer.

Angiosarcoma: Angiosarcomas are rare primary hepatic malignancies and are the most common malignant mesenchymal neoplasm. Angiosarcomas are typically not encapsulated and involve the liver diffusely. Ultrasonography demonstrates multiple, ill-defined hyperechoic lesions. On contrast-enhanced CT, angiosarcomas have marked contrast enhancement and may mimic hemangioma closely; however, if intraperitoneal hemorrhage is present, angiosarcoma is highly suspected. On MRI, angiosarcomas are hypointe nse with focal hyperintensity on T1-weighted images and heterointense on T2-weighted images.

Conclusion

Liver masses are a common clinical problem and especially so with the increased use of modern imaging modalities. The appropriate clinical management relies on an accurate diagnosis. A thorough clinical history, laboratory data, and liver imaging can provide the definitive diagnosis in the majority of patients (Fig. 2.3). Liver biopsy is reserved for select patients who are not candidates for resection, those in whom the diagnosis would preclude operative exploration, or when an exact diagnosis is necessary for treatment planning.

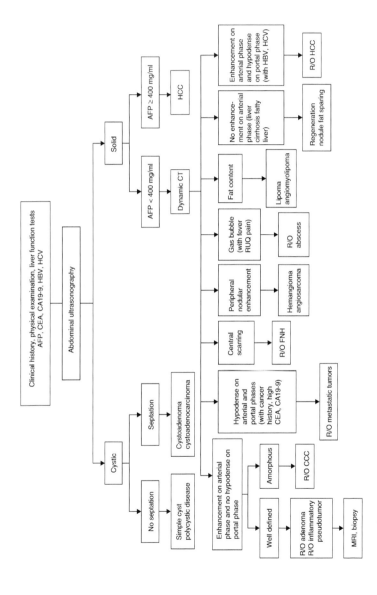

FIGURE 2.3. Differential diagnosis of the liver mass.

Selected Readings

Gibbs JF, Litwin AM, Kahlenberg MS (2004) Contemporary management of benign liver tumors. Surg Clin N Am 84:463–480

Hammerstingl RM, Schwarz W, Vogl TJ (2003) Contrast agents. In: Vogl TJ, Lencioni R, Hammerstingl RM, Bartolozzi C (eds) Magnetic resonance imaging in liver disease. Georg Thieme Verlag, Stuttgart/New York, pp 45–91

Lee WC, Jeng LB, Chen MF (2002) Estimation of prognosis after hepatectomy for hepatocellular carcinoma. Br J Surg 89:311–316

Lee WC, Jeng LB, Chen MF (2000) Hepatectomy for hepatitis B-, hepatitis C-, and dual hepatitis B-and C-related hepatocellular carcinoma in Taiwan. J Hepatobiliary Pancreat Surg 7:265–269

Yeh CN, Lee WC, Chen MF, Tsay PK (2003) Predictors of long-term disease-free survival after resection of hepatocellular carcinoma: two decades of experience at Chang-Gung Memorial Hospital. Ann Surg Oncol 10:916–921

3
Benign Hepatic Neoplasms

Juan Hepp

Pearls and Pitfalls

- Hepatic lesions are frequently identified incidentally on imaging performed for other purposes.
- With the exception of large lesions, benign hepatic neoplasms are typically asymptomatic.
- With current high quality imaging, it is possible to differentiate the majority of hepatic neoplasms as benign or malignant.
- Resection of indeterminant, worrisome lesions is generally preferred over biopsy.
- Hepatic hemangioma is the most common, solid lesion found in the liver.
- Focal nodular hyperplasia (FNH) does not require resection, but at the least, initial follow-up imaging is recommended.

Introduction

The more frequent use of imaging studies of the abdomen, especially ultrasonography (US), has lead to frequent consultation because of the finding of an (often) asymptomatic hepatic lesion. The lesion can be solid or cystic, benign or malignant, or a primary or secondary neoplasm. These patients should be evaluated with thorough clinical history and

K.I. Bland et al. (eds.), *Liver and Biliary Surgery*,
DOI 10.1007/978-1-84996-429-6_3,
© Springer-Verlag London Limited 2011

TABLE 3.1. Benign liver tumors.

Origin	Denomination
Epithelial	
Hepatocellular	Focal nodular hyperplasia
	Hepatocellular adenoma
	Regenerative nodule
Cholangiocellular	Simple cyst
	Biliary cystadenoma
	Biliary adenoma
Mesenchymal	
Endothelial	Hemangioma
	Hemangioendothelioma

appropriate diagnostic studies. The most frequent benign solid and cystic lesions of the liver are listed in Table 3.1.

Hemangioma

The incidence of hemangiomas is approximately 5% in adults and 7% in autopsies, and they are the most frequently identified lesion in the liver. Hemangiomas are more frequent in women and adults. The most usual form are the capillary hemangiomas, typically small, followed by the cavernous hemangiomas, which can reach considerable size and are more likely to cause symptoms. Hemangiomas (Fig. 3.1a) usually have characteristic features on imaging that allow a confident, non-invasive diagnosis (see Chapter 2). Grossly, these lesions are well delineated, and their macroscopic aspect is easy to recognize by the surgeon (Fig. 3.1b). The hemangioma sometimes generates a fibrous plane in contact with the liver, facilitating its enucleation.

Symptoms arise typically from compression of adjacent organs or rapid enlargement due to intratumoral bleeding or thrombosis. Rupture with bleeding into the peritoneum is exceedingly rare, but when this occurs, the associated mortality

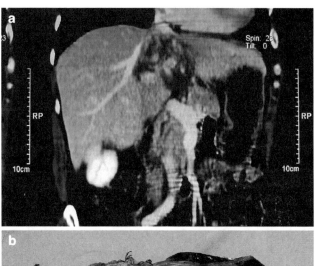

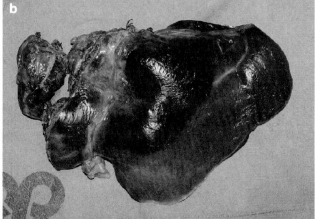

FIGURE 3.1. Central cavernous hemangioma. (**a**) CT: note compression of hepatic veins. (**b**) Left liver resection that includes the cavernous hemangioma and a smaller neighboring hemangioma.

is very high. Patient stabilization is vital in these cases, and different methods can be used to obtain some stabilization, including arteriographic embolization, hepatic artery ligation, and perihepatic packing to control the hemorrhage and allow a resection under more appropriate conditions. The rarity of spontaneous rupture does not justify a preventive hepatic resection of even large but asymptomatic hemangiomas.

The literature mentions frequently the term "giant" hemangioma with no consensus regarding the size of the lesion. Hemangiomas with a diameter >4 cm are described as giant hemangiomas but do not imply any special therapeutic implications. The mass effect of large hemangiomas 20 cm or larger may produce discomfort, malaise, or obstructive symptoms and may be palpable on physical examination. Clear correlation of the symptoms with the lesion should guide the appropriateness of operative intervention. Laboratory work-up is typically normal, even for large hemangiomas. The Kasabach-Merritt syndrome, most commonly described in patients with thrombocytopenia and consumption coagulopathy secondary to skin and spleen hemangiomas, may occur rarely with liver hemangiomas. Very few cases have been described, and the treatment is enucleation or liver transplantation.

Imaging studies beginning with US usually make the diagnosis. Fortunately, good quality US and its adequate interpretation is usually sufficient for the diagnosis of hemangioma. Hyperechogenicity with well-defined borders is typical, and if Doppler exam is added, a greater vascular flow is appreciated easily. Typical CT findings suggesting hemangioma include a hypodense lesion in comparison with the surrounding liver parenchyma. After injecting intravenous contrast, the lesion fills irregularly from the periphery reaching the center after a few minutes. The enhanced lesion persists longer than the rest of the liver (Fig. 3.1). This finding is typical of hemangioma. The specificity of MRI exceeds that of CT in the diagnosis of hemangioma. Disadvantages of MRI, however, include cost, availability, expertise, and contraindications in persons with pacemakers or metallic prostheses, and it may require sedation in claustrophobic patients. Both methods allow simultaneous evaluation of the remainder of the abdomen as well. MRI offers the advantage of use in patients with allergy to contrast media. Hemangiomas are characteristically hyperintense on the T2-weighted images; after administration of gadolinium, a peripheral filling lesion similar to CT findings is noted. Although hepatic scintigraphy with ^{99m}Tc-labeled red blood cells has diagnostic merit, this study has been supplanted by the previously described imaging methods. Selective arteriography of the liver shows a corkscrew aspect of the vessels and a cotton-like filling, both of which are very characteristic. This method is almost never required because of its cost and invasive nature.

Biopsy of lesions suspicious for hemangioma is generally not advised due to the risk of complications and failure to exclude definitively a neoplasm. A biopsy of any focal liver lesion is useful only if it will change the therapeutic plan; otherwise, the lesion should be observed or resected.

For asymptomatic hemangiomas, once a confident diagnosis has been made, the therapeutic approach for the vast majority of these cases is periodic observation. Yearly follow-up of the lesion with US may demonstrate that the lesion does not grow and does not develop changes within the lesion. Complications developing from an asymptomatic lesion during follow-up are very unusual, not predictable, and do not justify resection.

Rarely, one may see a hemangioma that enlarges through the years, for instance, during pregnancy (Fig. 3.2).

The indications for resection of hemangioma include symptomatic lesions or patients in whom the diagnosis is uncertain. Patient concerns, performance status, and other medical conditions also impact the decision for operative intervention. Some patients with a large hemangioma have been advised erroneously to undergo extirpation of the hemangioma because of

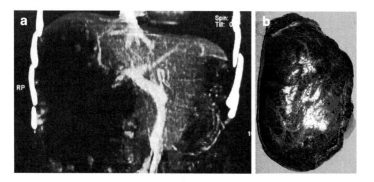

FIGURE 3.2. Large right hepatic hemangioma that enlarged rapidly during pregnancy. (**a**) CT; (**b**) resected hemangioma.

symptoms not related to the neoplasm. In a very anxious patient in whom the lesion is easily resectable, the operative risk is relatively low, and if the patient understands the risks, resection may be appropriate. The majority of symptomatic, resected, or complicated hemangiomas are larger than 10 cm. The management of hemangiomas that measure ≥15 cm is controversial in otherwise asymptomatic patients. It seems reasonable to observe them periodically and carefully, and if there is any evidence of growth or symptomatology, to resect them.

Operative resection involves enucleation or formal anatomic resection, depending on the location and relationship to portal branches and hepatic veins. Operative approach, laparotomy, and laparoscopic approaches depend on the location, size, and characteristics of the lesion. Planning the resection will also depend on intra-operative findings. Sometimes a simple enucleation of a hemangioma that "hangs" from the liver will be possible; in other patients, the hemangioma may be a deep lesion that requires a surgeon expert in hepatic resections. Often a fibrous plane exists between the hemangioma and the hepatic tissue that facilitates a safe and easy enucleation. An especially useful tool is the ultrasonic dissector that facilitates enucleation of the hemangioma. Because hemangiomas are benign lesions, it is not necessary to resect margins of healthy liver. Full visualization and mobilization of the liver with early control of the vascular pedicles facilitates the resection. On occasion, a dominant hepatic artery or an arterial branch that feeds preferentially the lesion can be found.

Preemptive transvascular embolization of the hemangioma is not justified based on the low risk of spontaneous hemorrhage but has been very useful in the management of ruptured hemangiomas. It is not uncommon to find neighboring smaller hemangiomas when resecting a large one; however, they require no intervention, because they have an exceedingly small risk of becoming symptomatic. Postoperative complications are rare and are the same as those found in any hepatic resection.

Focal Nodular Hyperplasia (FNH)

FNH was first described in 1958. This lesion believed to be hormone-dependent is much more frequent in young women and has been related to the use of oral contraceptives. FNH can reach considerable size, yet most are asymptomatic and found only incidentally on an imaging procedure for another complaint. When symptoms do appear, they are secondary to its mass effect. Malignant degeneration or hemorrhage has not been described. FNH is a macroscopically well-defined lesion without a capsule arising within otherwise normal hepatic tissue. The lesion appears more pale than normal liver, has prominent vessels on its surface, and presents a somewhat lobulated aspect, with a firm, rubbery consistency (Fig. 3.3a). Frequently, a central radial scar consisting of a vascularized fibrous septum is seen characteristically on imaging studies. Histologically, this lesion suggests a regenerative nodule with a predominance of Küpffer cells and biliary duct hyperplasia, thus differentiating FNH histologically from adenomas. Differentiating FNH from adenoma preoperatively on imaging studies, however, may prove challenging. Biliary scintigraphy with radiolabeled sulfur colloid shows a prominent uptake by the abundant Küpffer cells into the FNH, thereby allowing the differentiation from adenoma. Ultrasonography shows an echogenic lesion but only occasionally having the "characteristic" central, vascularized scar. CTandMRIshowa homogeneous,vascularized lesion and, when present, outlining a radial central scar with a "cartwheel" aspect (Fig. 3.4) that differentiates FNH from adenoma; however, smaller lesions usually lack the features. Arteriography is not recommended, but when done will show a well-vascularized lesion and, when present, the central, vascularized scar. Usually one of these techniques will permit a confident diagnosis. On occasion, however, a small lesion (<5 cm) can be seen in a central location. Biopsy is not recommended, because it will usually be inconclusive. In patients without substantive risk factors like cirrhosis or chronic viral infection, follow-up imaging in 3–6 months

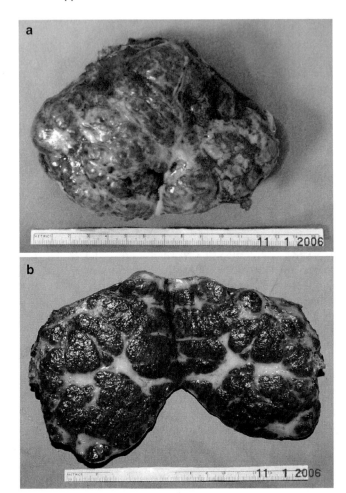

FIGURE 3.3. Focal nodular hyperplasia. (**a**) External macroscopic view. Note uneven surface. (**b**) Cut surface of resected tumor.

seems the best approach; if the lesion remains unchanged over time, a benign lesion seems most likely. Growth in size, however, warrants an aggressive approach. For the peripherally located, small lesions, a laparoscopic wedge excision may be the best approach unless FNH is highly suspected, in which case follow-up imaging surveillance seems best.

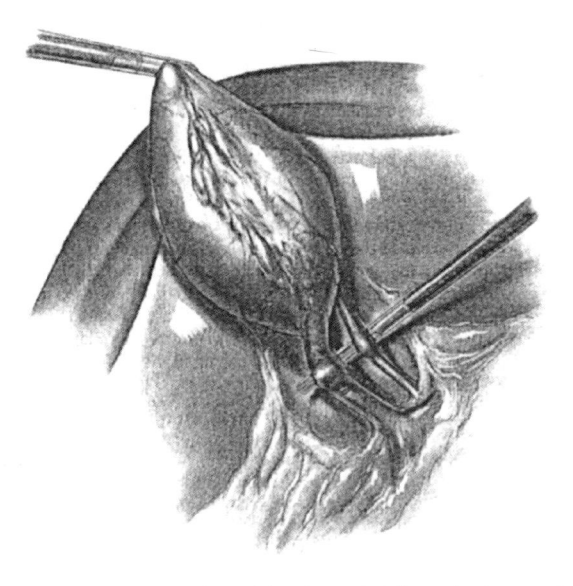

FIGURE 13.2. Conclusive identification of the cystic duct and artery by demonstration of the "critical view of safety". Only two structures (the cystic duct and artery) are connected to the lowest part of the gallbladder when its attachment to the liver bed has been freed From Strasberg SM, Hertl M, Soper NJ: An analysis of the problem of biliairy injury during laparoscopic cholecystectomy. J Am Coll Surg 1995;180:101–125. Reproduced with permission from the Journal of the American College of Surgeons.

anatomy correctly and aids the identification of BDI should it occur. Recognition of injury at the time of LC improves greatly the outcome associated with early repair. IOC is cost effective, can be performed relatively quickly and should be taught to all surgical trainees.

Conversion from Laparoscopic to Open Cholecystectomy

Laparoscopic cholecystectomy should be converted to an open procedure without hesitation if there is any concern regarding bile duct injury or if the biliary anatomy cannot be

TABLE 13.1. Technical points from the Guidelines for the Clinical Application of Laparoscopic Biliary Tract Surgery from the Society of American Gastrointestinal and Endoscopic Surgeons.

- The cystic duct should be identified at its junction with the gallbladder

- Traction of the gallbladder infundibulum should be lateral rather than cephalad

- Meticulous dissection of the cystic duct and cystic artery is essential

- All energy sources may cause occult injury

- Biliary tract imaging should be applied liberally to identify surgically important anomalies, clarify difficult anatomy, and detect common bile duct stones

- The surgeon should convert to open operation for irresolvable technical difficulties or anatomic uncertainties oranomalies, especially in cases of acute cholecystitis

from complete excision of the extrahepatic biliary tree associated with division of the right hepatic artery.

Intraoperative Cholangiography in the Prevention of Bile Duct Injury

The role of intra operative cholangiography (IOC) in the prevention of BDI remains controversial; no randomized control trials have been carried out to assess its role in avoiding BDI since it is likely that a very large number of patients would be required for such a study given the relatively low incidence of injury. However, there is good evidence from large population based studies that supports a role for IOC in helping to prevent BDI. Flum and colleagues examined the outcome of 1.5 million laparoscopic cholecystectomies and demonstrated that not performing an IOC was associated with a two-fold increased risk of BDI. It is vital to appreciate that the use of IOC does not obviate the need for meticulous dissection and careful identification of the anatomy, but when used liberally, it is a useful adjunct to help identify the

Symptomatic cholelithiasis: For symptomatic patients, cholecystectomy is the only proven treatment which can eliminate symptoms of biliary colic and prevent complications. Once symptoms develop, much more than 50% of patients will have recurrent symptoms. The worry, of course, is that these patients will develop a serious complication.

Acute cholecystitis: Obstruction of the cystic duct produces gallbladder distension, irritation of the mucosa with potential wall ischemia, inflammation, and potentially necrosis. Ischemic necrosis of the gallbladder wall is the result of the gallbladder distension with eventual obstruction and thrombosis of cystic blood vessels. Ischemia and necrosis may lead to gallbladder perforation with either an adjacent liver abscess, a walled-off pericholecystic abscess, or less commonly, free intra-abdominal perforation with secondary bile peritonitis.

Diagnosis of acute cholecystitis should be suspected in patients with a history of biliary colic, a clinical presentation of intense biliary colic pain, and a physical examination that reveals tenderness on the right upper quadrant, associated with fever, a positive Murphy sign, and a palpable, tender gallbladder. Clinical jaundice is rare, although an increased serum bilirubin of >1.5 mg/dl is not uncommon.

Same admission cholecystectomy is the treatment of choice among patients with acute cholecystitis unless contraindications for operative intervention exist or the risk of an operation in the acute setting exceeds alternative options. Once the diagnosis is made, cholecystectomy should not be delayed, because the progressive inflammation can make the operation more difficult. Laparoscopic cholecystectomy is the preferred operative approach in acute cholecystitis, although difficulty with surrounding inflammation and delineating anatomy increase the conversion rate to open cholecystectomy over patients with symptomatic cholelithiasis undergoing elective cholecystectomy. Some surgeons will advocate a delayed cholecystectomy in patients with acute cholecystitis of more than 5–10 days' duration who are improving. Often the cholecystitis will resolve, and an elective cholecystectomy 5 weeks later will have a greater likelihood of being accomplished laparoscopically.

and in experienced hands has a sensitivity comparable to that of endoscopic retrograde cholangio-pancreatography (ERCP). Although advantages include being non-invasive, MRCP is expensive, not widely available, requires radiologic expertise in its interpretation, and does not allow the opportunity for simultaneous treatment of choledocholithiasis.

Treatment

In patients with cholelithiasis, laparoscopic cholecystectomy is the treatment of choice. Many studies have demonstrated decreased pain, shorter hospital stay, earlier return to work, and decreased complication rates of a laparoscopic compared with open cholecystectomy. Conversely, bile duct injury is increased somewhat with laparoscopic approaches.

Asymptomatic cholelithiasis: It has been estimated that in the United States about 1% per year of asymptomatic patients will develop symptoms or other complications related to cholelithiasis with observation. Therefore, in the United States, cholecystectomy is generally not recommended for asymptomatic patients. In contrast, in countries such as Chile, the incidence of developing symptomatic cholelithiasis is increased. Up to 12% of asymptomatic patients develop gallstone-related symptoms during a 2-year follow up, 17% after 4 years, and 25% after 10-year follow-up. Only 3% of these patients, however, develop serious associated complications (acute cholecystitis, choledocholithiasis, or acute pancreatitis). In Chile, Bolivia and certain parts of Northern India, for instance, there is a very high incidence of gallbladder cancer, which is associated with cholelithiasis in 90% of patients. Therefore, cholecystectomy is offered for most patients with cholelithiasis, irrespective of symptoms, to prevent the development of gallbladder cancer. Indications for the operative treatment of asymptomatic patients with cholelithiasis should, therefore, be based on patient clinical data, personal, family, and ethnic history.

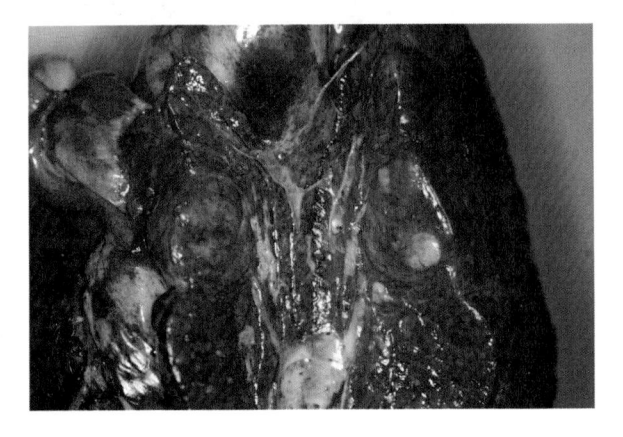

FIGURE 9.3. Numerous tiny yellowish nodules. This is the diffuse type of HCC of a patient who was planned for liver transplantation. Because of the finding, liver transplantation was aborted.

HCC tends to invade luminal structures within the liver. Thus, branches of the portal vein, hepatic vein, bile duct, and lymphatics maybe involved, with tumor spread from the terminal branches toward the major branch. The portal vein is involved most commonly by local invasion (Fig. 9.4). The tumor grows in the portal vein against the bloodstream. When segmental branches are reached, tumor fragments are dislodged, and emboli are disseminated to the adjacent liver segments. Such mode of spread accounts for the appearance of satellite nodules in the liver segments adjacent to the main neoplasm or contralateral liver when the bifurcation of the portal vein is invaded by HCC. Due to invasion into the hepatic vein, the lung is the most common site of extrahepatic spread. Peritoneal metastasis is unusual unless there is previous spontaneous rupture of HCC or puncture of a superficial HCC by biopsy needle.

The prognosis of HCC can be gauged by the histologic features. Neoplasms with evidence of invasion, e.g. lymphovascular permeation, liver invasion, invasion across tumor capsule, bile duct invasion, or microsatellite lesions, are associated with poor outcome. In contrast, solitary tumors without vascular invasion are associated with a relatively good prognosis.

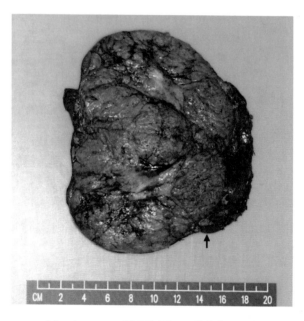

FIGURE 9.1. Massive type HCC. The adjoining nodule (arrow) represents spread from the primary neoplasm.

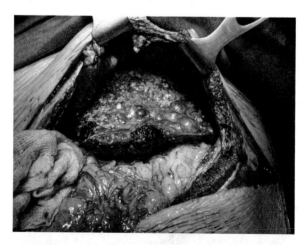

FIGURE 9.2. Nodular type HCC in a liver explant.

identified with certainty. Prolonged inappropriate attempts at defining the anatomy should be avoided. If the operating field is not clear during laparoscopic dissection because of anomalous anatomy, adhesions or bleeding, then conversion may be a safer approach rather than risk injury. Given that the modern surgeon may be much more familiar with the laparoscopic than open approach to cholecystectomy, it is important to appreciate when conversion is necessary, that the operative conditions may be challenging as a result of distorted anatomy and inflamed tissues. It is therefore important that surgeons undertaking laparoscopic cholecystectomy are proficient in the open approach. Importantly, if dissection in the area of Calot's triangle cannot be undertaken safely, the surgeon may consider a fundus first or retrograde dissection of the fundus of the gallbladder from the liver bed. However, it is essential to identify the correct plane of dissection since the layer of fibrous tissue known as the cystic plate may be densely adherent to gallbladder and liver bed. This tissue is part of the perihilar system of fibrous tissue and attaches onto the anterior surface of the right portal pedicle. Dissection deep to the plate may therefore risk injury to any peripheral bile duct and the origin of the middle hepatic vein in the liver bed but more importantly to the right hepatic duct or artery if this cystic plate is fused to the right portal pedicle. In such circumstances, it is wiser to undertake a subtotal cholecystectomy leaving the posterior wall of the gallbladder in situ rather than risk inadvertent injury to the structures in the right portal pedicle. In the acute setting, it may be prudent to accept that cholecystostomy may represent the safer immediate management of the inflamed gallbladder.

Classification of Bile Duct Injury

A number of different classification systems of BDI have been described (Table 13.2) These schemes have a number of limitations in that they are not inclusive of some of the most serious variants of BDI and also have inappropriate inclusions.

TABLE 13.2. Summary of proposed classification of bile duct injuries (Connor and Garden, 2006).

Reference	Bismuth 1982	Strasberg et al. 1995	Stewart et al. 2004	Keulemans et al. 1998	Csendes et al. 2001	Schmidt et al. 2004
Cystic duct or terminal biliary radical leak		A		A		A
Bile leak from CBD/CHD without tissue loss		D	I	B1	I,II	C
Bile leak with tissue loss from CHD/CBD			II	B1	III	D
Bile leak from right hepatic duct (posterior sector)		C	IV	B2		
Transection or occlusion of CBD or CHD			III	D	III	B or D
Strictures						
CBD stricture						E
CHD stricture >2 cm	I	E1	III	C	III,IV	E
CHD stricture <2 cm	II	E2	III	C	III,IV	E
Hilar stricture but confluence intact	III	E3	III	C	III,IV	E
Hilar stricture with disruption of confluence	IV	E4	III	C	III,IV	E
Obstructed right posterior hepatic duct with or without CBD/CHD stricture.		V	B/E5	IV	C	E

None of these describes one of the most serious injuries which involve the excision of the extra hepatic biliary tree with separation of the right and left ducts (Fig. 13.3). A further important omission from these schemes is the absence of adequate criteria to describe a concomitant vascular injury to either the arterial, or portal systems (Fig. 13.4). Such vascular injuries can occur in association with BDI and are associated with a poor outcome following repair. Inappropriate inclusions in these schemes include bile leaks from the cystic duct and terminal biliary radicals which should properly be considered as complications of cholecystectomy, rather than bile duct injuries per se. This distinction is necessary because it is exceptional for such complications to produce lasting morbidity or require specialist repair unless the signs of bile leak are ignored in the patient whose recovery from laparoscopic surgery is slow. These classification schemes have helped stratify BDIs for the purpose of identifying prognostic outcomes in descriptive studies, but they must be considered along with further important prognostic factors including the mode of presentation, previous attempts at repair, the presence of sepsis and the clinical condition of the patient.

Diagnosis and Assessment of BDI

BDI must be recognized early if the consequent repair is to be successful. Key to early diagnosis is a high level of suspicion both during the operative phase and in the post operative period. Up to 90% of injuries are not identified during the initial surgery. It would be expected that the patient recovering from uneventful cholecystectomy would be ready for discharge within hours of operation. In the post operative period, any patient who remains unwell 24 h following surgery should be investigated to exclude a diagnosis of BDI. The indicators of injury will vary depending on the exact nature of the injury but jaundice, abdominal pain, peritonitis or sepsis may all result from damage to the biliary tree. The

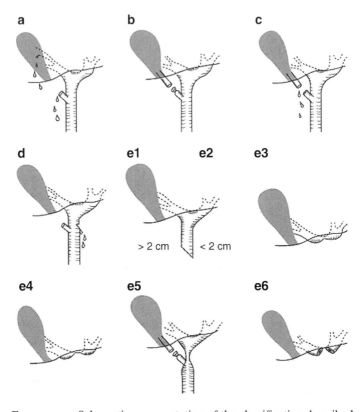

FIGURE 13.3. Schematic representation of the classification described by Strasberg and colleagues. (**a**) Bile leak from cystic duct stump or minor biliary radical in gallbladder fossa. (**b**) Occluded right posterior sectoral duct. (**c**) Bile leak from divided right posterior sectoral duct. (**d**) Bile leak from main bile duct without major tissue loss. (**e1**) Transected main bile duct with a stricture more than 2 cm from the hilus. (**e2**) Transected main bile duct with a stricture less than 2 cm from the hilus. (**e3**) Stricture of the hilus with right and left ducts in communication. (**e4**) Stricture of the hilus with separation of the right and left ducts. (**e5**) Stricture of the main bile duct and the posterior sectoral duct. (**e6**) Complete excision of the extrahepatic ducts involving the confluence (this injury is not described in Strasberg's classification. From Connor S, Garden OJ. Bile duct injury in the era of laparoscopic cholecystectomy. Br J Surg 2006;93:158–168. ©2006 British Journal of Surgery Society Ltd. Reproduced with permission. Permission is granted by John Wiley & Sons Ltd on Behalf of the BJSS Ltd.).

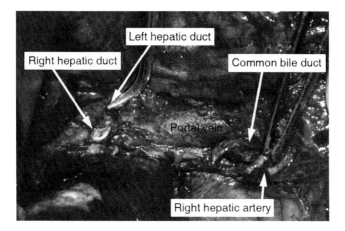

FIGURE 13.4. Operative view one of the most serious injuries (E6) which involves damage to the right hepatic artery which has been clipped and divided, with excision of the extra hepatic biliary tree resulting in separation of the right and left ducts.

patient who still has a requirement for significant amounts of analgesia within 12 h of surgery and who has abnormal liver function tests should be assessed carefully even in the absence of abdominal signs. Evidence of a systemic inflammatory response should not be attributed to other possible complications until the diagnosis of intra-abdominal bile leak has been excluded. The diagnosis of BDI is often delayed by up to 2 weeks, by which stage the option of early repair may be lost. Initial investigations should include liver function tests and abdominal imaging. Ultrasonography (US) may not always be sensitive in confirming the presence of an intra-abdominal complication. Collections of fluid can be found in the GB fossa in one in five patients who have undergone LC but should not be dismissed lightly in the presence of adverse clinical signs or biochemical abnormalities. Computed tomography (CT) should be performed preferentially or if US is equivocal as it has a higher sensitivity than US for demonstrating intra abdominal collections and their extent. Furthermore, a contrast enhanced CT scan may alert to the possibility of an associated injury to the right hepatic artery by demonstrating a perfusion abnormality. Collections of fluid should be aspirated or drained by the percutaneous route or by laparoscopy or laparotomy as the presence of bile in the peritoneal cavity can lead quickly to peritonitis and be more difficult to eradicate. If the aspirate contains bile, it should be assumed there has been a bile duct injury and a high quality cholangiogram should be performed. Magnetic resonance cholangiopancreatography (MRCP) is the first test of choice (Fig. 13.5). If the MRCP demonstrates a leak from an accessory duct, from the cystic duct stump, or if there are gall stones in the CBD, endoscopic retrograde cholangio-pancreatography (ERCP) should be performed. If a major duct has been injured, ERCP is not considered helpful and may lead to a delay in subsequent definitive treatment.

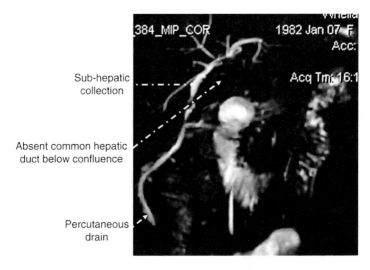

FIGURE 13.5. MRCP demonstrating a bile leak from immediately below the confluence of the right and left hepatic ducts with flow of bile into a subhepatic collection. At operation, it was evident that the main bile duct had been excised along with the gallbladder. A drain lies within a collection beneath the gallbladder bed.

The diagnosis of BDI mandates immediate referral to a hepatobiliary surgeon. Whether the injury is identified during surgery, or at any time in the post operative period, the operating surgeon should not attempt repair since attempted repair by the injuring surgeon is associated with an increased risk of morbidity and mortality. It is accepted that a non-specialist surgeon attempting BDI repair is more likely to achieve a poorer result, prolong the postoperative stay of the patient and increase markedly the risk of serious complication and death.

Following referral to an experienced hepatobiliary surgeon, further assessment may require imaging of the arterial and portal vasculature, which may be injured in up to a third of cases, using MR or CT angiography. On occasion, unrelieved biliary obstruction may be associated with the development of liver abscess which will require prolonged antibiotic therapy and drainage of substantial collections and of the biliary tree. If BDI is diagnosed late, following the development of a biliary stricture, then the function of the obstructed liver should be determined, with liver biopsy if necessary since hepatic fibrosis can occur a year without adequate management. Atrophy of the liver may be evident if there is impaired drainage to one part of the liver or vascular compromise.

Management of Bile Duct Injury

The way in which bile duct injury is managed is determined by a number of factors including the delay between injury and diagnosis, the degree of intra abdominal sepsis and the type of the injury.

Immediate Repair Following Intra Operative Diagnosis

During surgery, either the leakage of bile or an abnormal cholangiogram may raise the possibility of a BDI and the opinion of an experienced hepatobiliary surgeon should be sought, as this has been shown to increase the success of consequent repair. If this is not possible, large non suction drains should be placed close to the injured duct to ensure drainage of bile, and the patient should be transferred to an appropriate center. If a bile leak can be attributed definitively to an accessory duct, consideration can be given to its ligation but the operating surgeon should be aware that obstructive segmental cholangitis, hepatic abscess and prolonged biliary fistula may result. The injuring surgeon should not attempt repair of a significant bile duct injury since inappropriate attempts may increase the severity of the injury. If there is a bile leak from the region of the porta hepatis or proximal GB fossa, an operative cholangiogram at this stage may not be helpful as forceful cannulation may increase the severity of the injury. A major injury to the CBD is likely to require repair by means of a hepaticojejunostomy.

Early Repair Following Diagnosis in the Post Operative Period

If BDI is identified early in the post operative period, the priorities of treatment before any reconstructive surgery can be planned include the drainage of intra abdominal collections, the establishment of a controlled biliary fistula and the treatment of sepsis. The opinion of a hepatobiliary surgeon should be sought promptly and the patient should be transferred to an appropriate center if necessary. Early referral is vital following bile duct injury since there exists only a short window of 1–2 weeks during which BDI can be repaired (6) with the expectation of a shorter duration of treatment and subsequently improved quality of life. Beyond this period the likelihood of such a favorable outcome falls as a result of sepsis and a major inflammatory response. In this situation, it would be our practice to delay repair for a minimum of 3 months. Even if bile duct injury is recognized within the early postoperative period, the possible presence of concomitant vascular injury, significant diathermy injury or established sepsis, is likely to compromise successful anastomosis and long-term outcome.

Delayed Repair

If attempts at definitivetreatment aretobedelayed as aconsequenceoflatediagnosis of injury or the criteria for a successful anastomosis are not met, the priorities in the interim are aimed at controlling the leakage of bile, treatment of sepsis and the provision of nutritional support. Localized intraabdominal collections can usually be drained percutaneously although multiple loculi of bile may be better managed by open lavage and the placement of drains. Consequent proximal control with the placement of a percutaneous transhepatic external biliary drain, if possible, may allow abdominal drains to be withdrawn thereby reducing inflammation at the site of injury and allowing the tissues to mature. Maintaining adequate nutrition during the period prior to delayed repair will increase the likelihood of a successful outcome. Bile re-feeding may be necessary if the patient has an external biliary fistula for a prolonged period.

Surgical Approach to the Repair of Bile Duct Injury

Primary Closure

Partial defects in the bile duct without significant devascularization or trauma to surrounding tissue are uncommon but should be repaired with primary closure using fine absorbable interrupted sutures with the placement of drains. The placement of a T tube may be associated with a higher stricture rate than without as has been shown in liver transplantation and it would be our practice to avoid their use but to employ abdominal drainage to avoid further intra-abdominal contamination.

Primary repair of a complete bile duct transection has been reported but it may be difficult to appreciate the extent of the injury to the damaged duct and it seems to carry a significant rate of failure in many reported series. It would not be the preferred approach by the majority of surgeons experienced in the management of bile duct injury.

Hepaticojejunostomy

Major BDIs should be repaired with a hepaticojejunostomy Roux-en-Y and there is no place for hepatico-duodenostomy or direct choledocho-choledochostomy since the latter procedure, in particular, appears to be associated with a higher risk of stricture. The most common long-term complication of hepaticojejunostomy is anastomotic stricture and so it is vital that this is effected using healthy well vascularized tissue in a non-infected environment. In both the acute and late setting, we advocate a "left duct approach" in which the left hepatic duct is opened longitudinally for 1–3 cm, allowing for a wide anastomosis to jejunum. Following recent injury, the left duct can usually be identified easily by probing the open bile duct and is incised along its anterior wall at the base of segment IV, taking care to avoid inadvertent injury to the arterial branch to this segment and which may limit the length of the biliary stoma (Fig. 13.6). In the delayed setting, the duct may require to be exposed by lowering the hilar plate with a Cavitron Ultrasonic Aspirator (CUSA). This maneuver combined with opening the fibrosed gallbladder bed and the often adherent left and quadrate lobes provides excellent access to the left duct. A single layer anastomosis fashioned with absorbable sutures to healthy, non-inflamed or scarred tissue is most liable to result in a satisfactory outcome. Opening the left duct longitudinally creates a wide anastomosis which would normally incorporate the left and right segmental ducts. It would not be our preference to undertake this repair with transanastomotic stenting although others feel that abetter result can be obtained in their hands using such an approach. In complex injuries, it is normally more difficult to achieve a satisfactory anastomosis to the intrahepatic right duct access

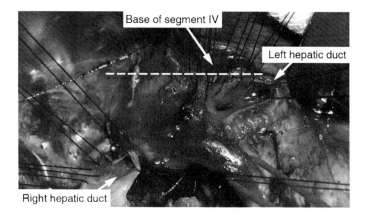

FIGURE 13.6. Operative view demonstrating exposure of the right and left hepatic ducts following an E6 injury sustained during laparoscopic cholecystectomy.

to which may involve extensive dissection within the hepatic parenchyma to expose the right intrahepatic pedicle. In this unusual situation where such access is difficult or if there is associated injury to the right hepatic artery or atrophy of the right liver, it may be prudent to undertake a right hepatectomy. A more favorable long-term outcome may be achieved by accepting sacrifice of the right hemiliver when a satisfactory and secure anastomosis can be realized easily to the left hepatic duct.

Role of Endoscopic Treatment in the Management of BDI

Endoscopic retrograde cholangiography (ERC) in combination with stenting or sphincterotomy is the appropriate procedure for the treatment of complications such as a bile leak from the cystic duct or a terminal biliary radical identified in the post operative period. It must be appreciated, however, that the diagnosis of a bile leak in the early postoperative period also requires consideration for the need to effect adequate drainage of the peritoneal cavity. Diagnostic or therapeutic ERC should not be considered as a definitive treatment for biliary contamination or peritonitis. ERC may also be appropriate for suspected small incomplete defects in the side of the bile duct but published reports suggest that endoscopic management remains inferior to surgery. Endoscopic or radiological treatment of major bile duct injuries such as biliary strictures includes balloon dilatation and the placement of biliary stents. Such approaches are generally again considered to be less successful than surgery, although may have a place in the treatment of the patient in whom surgery is not possible or as an adjunct to surgery in certain challenging situations. Definitive endoscopic treatment of major bile duct injury should only be undertaken within a specialist service with experience in the management of bile duct injury, or following discussion with the specialist team. Prolonged attempts at managing bile duct injury endoscopically risk introducing the specter of recurrent biliary sepsis and secondary biliary cirrhosis.

Long Term Outcome Following Repair for Bile Duct Injury

Complications, particularly anastomotic stricture are not uncommon following hepaticojejunostomy for bile duct injury and may occur many years after apparent successful surgery. Therefore, such patients should be followed up for a prolonged period of up to ten years to exclude the development of biliary obstructive symptoms and to ensure that liver function tests do not demonstrate evidence of cholestasis. Recurrent jaundice and biliary sepsis may occur in a third of patients after apparent successful BDI repair. Poor outcome following reconstructive surgery is more common when referral to a specialist center has been delayed, with increasing severity of injury and if multiple attempts at repair have been made previously. Nonetheless, with careful planning and management of injuries, a satisfactory outcome can be achieved in 70–80% of patients.

Despite an apparent satisfactory and anatomical result following appropriate referral and repair, it has been shown that, these patients may go on to experience a poor quality of life. Long-term follow-up studies have shown that endoscopic treatment and duration of treatment prior to referral were associated with an unfavorable quality of life. Several studies have demonstrated that the psychological impact is often underestimated particularly for those patients who have had a prolonged period of treatment and in whom medical litigation is prolonged.

Selected Readings

Bismuth H (1982) Postoperative strictures of the bile duct. In: Blumgart LH (ed) The bilary tract. Churchill Livingstone, Edinburgh, pp. 209–218

Connor S, Garden OJ (2006) Bile duct injury in the era of laparoscopic cholecystectomy. Br J Surg 93:158–168

Csendes A, Navarrete C, Burdiles P, Yarmuch J (2001) Treatment of common bile duct injuries during laparoscopic cholecystectomy: endoscopic and surgical management. World J Surg 25:1346–1351

Flum DR, Dellinger EP, Cheadle A, Chan L, Koepsell T (2003) Intraoperative cholangiography and risk of common bile duct injury during cholecystectomy. JAMA 289:1639–1644

Hunter JG (1991) Avoidance of bile duct injury during laparoscopic cholecystectomy. Am J Surg 162:71–76

Keulemans YC, Bergman JJ, de Wit LT, Rauws EA, Huibregtse K, Tytgat GN, et al. (1998) Improvement in the management of bile duct injuries? J Am Coll Surg 187:246–254

Schmidt SC, Settmacher U, Langrehr JM, Neuhaus P (2004) Management and outcome of patients with combined bile duct and hepatic arterial injuries after laparoscopic cho-lecystectomy. Surgery 135:613–618

Society of American Gastrointestinal Endoscopic Surgeons (SAGES) (2002) www.sages.org Guidelines for the clinical application of laparoscopic biliary tract surgery. The Society of American Gastrointestinal and Endoscopic Surgeons

Stewart L, Robinson TN, Lee CM, Liu K, Whang K, Way LW (2004) Right hepatic artery injury associated with laparoscopic bile duct injury: incidence, mechanism, and consequences. J Gastrointest Surg 8:523–530

Strasberg SM, Hertl M, Soper NJ (1995) An analysis of the problem of biliary injury during laparoscopic cholecys-tectomy. J Am Coll Surg 180:101–125

Thomson BN, Parks RW, Madhavan KK, Wigmore SJ, Garden OJ (2006) Early specialist repair of biliary injury. Br J Surg 93:216–220

14
Cholelithiasis

Luis A. Ibañez, Jean M. Butte, and Nicolás A. Devaud

Pearls and Pitfalls

- Cholelithiasis is asymptomatic in most patients.
- Abdominal ultrasonography is currently the best diagnostic tool, with a 95% sensitivity for gallstones.
- The presence of associated bile duct stones (choledocholithiasis) should be suspected through clinical signs such as jaundice and dark urine (bilirubinuria), together with radiologic and laboratory findings, such as bile duct dilation or increases in serum bilirubin concentration, alkaline phosphatase activity, or aspartate transaminase activity.
- In patients with a high suspicion of choledocholithiasis, MR cholangio-pancreatography (MRCP) provides a non-invasive, highly sensitive, diagnostic alternative.
- Most patients with asymptomatic cholelithiasis do not require cholecystectomy.
- Among symptomatic patients, laparoscopic cholecystectomy is the treatment of choice.
- Cholelithiasis is a major risk factor for gallbladder cancer.

K.I. Bland et al. (eds.), *Liver and Biliary Surgery*,
DOI 10.1007/978-1-84996-429-6_14,
© Springer-Verlag London Limited 2011

Introduction

Cholelithiasis is the presence of stones in the gallbladder. Gallstones in most cases consist of biliary cholesterol (80%), while about 20% consist of biliary pigments; the type of gallstone varies depending on sex, age, ethnic characteristics, and related hepatic and systemic disorders (e.g. cirrhosis, hemolysis). Therefore, differences in disease prevalence can be observed not only among different countries, but also among different regions of the same country. In the United States, an estimated 25 million adults have cholelithiasis, whereas in South American countries such as Chile, 20% of the adult male and 40–50% of the female population have cholelithiasis.

Cholelithiasis in the majority of patients is asymptomatic. Among these patients, the diagnosis is typically made incidentally on radiologic evaluations for unrelated symptoms or screening. Among symptomatic patients, the pain of biliary colic is the most common clinical presentation.

Ultrasonography is a highly sensitive, diagnostic exam (95%) with a positive predictive value of 97%. In addition to identifying stones, ultrasonography is useful in evaluation of other characteristics of the gallbladder (wall thickness, pericholecystic fluid, masses), intra-and extra-hepatic bile ducts, and adjacent organs in order to exclude associated choledocholithiasis and gallbladder neoplasms, given the association of the two conditions.

Choledocholithiasis should be suspected in those patients who present with jaundice and dark urine (bilirubinuria), extrahepatic bile duct dilation (>7 mm), or increases in serum conjugated bilirubin, alkaline phosphatase activity, or aspartate transaminase activity. In these patients, MR cholangiopancreatography (MRCP) is highly sensitive for the diagnosis of choledocholithiasis or any other bile duct changes. In patients in whom associated malignancies are suspected (gallbladder, pancreas, bile duct, or liver), contrast-enhanced abdominal computed tomography (CT) should be performed.

Laparoscopic cholecystectomy is the treatment of choice for symptomatic cholelithiasis. Among asymptomatic patients, however, there is no worldwide consensus with regard to the need for prophylactic cholecystectomy. The decision for cholecystectomy should be made considering personal and family history, other associated conditions, and possibly with regard to gallbladder cancer depending on ethnic race and geographic location.

In patients with choledocholithiasis, laparoscopic treatment options at the time of cholecystectomy may be considered depending on the experience of the surgical team. Typically, however, preoperative ERCP with extraction of choledocholithiasis is performed unless an open bile duct exploration is warranted; when the choledocholithiasis is discovered at the time of cholecystectomy, either a laparoscopic common bile duct exploration is carried out or treatment by endoscopic means is planned for the next day postoperatively.

Epidemiology

Many personal and ethnic factors are involved in the incidence and prevalence of cholelithiasis.

Sex: Among west Europeans, cholelithiasis is more prevalent in women (11%) than men (5%), while in the South American Chilean population, cholelithiasis is present in 40–50% of women and 20% of men. Estrogens have a defined role in hepatic cholesterol metabolism, increasing bile saturation, which in conjunction with changes in other biliary lipids, pigments, and the overall cholesterol saturation index predispose to the formation of gallstones.

Age: The prevalence of cholelithiasis increases markedly with age. Among subjects over 50 years of age, the prevalence of gallstones in the Western European population is 15% and in the South American population is 30% compared with a prevalence of only 2% in those between 18 and 31 years of age.

Obesity: Obese patients (BMI >30 kg/m^2) have a greater secretion of biliary cholesterol related to a greater production of cholesterol. Patients with BMI >25 kg/m^2 have a greater prevalence of cholelithiasis compared with those with BMI <25 kg/m^2 (13% vs. 7%). Interestingly, rapid or profound weight loss among obese patients, for instance, during starvation diets or after bariatric surgery, has also proven to be a risk factor for the development of cholelithiasis.

Pregnancy: Not only is pregnancy a well-known "risk factor" for cholelithiasis, multiparity increases the risk further. The hormonal and metabolic changes of pregnancy lead to an increased secretion and saturation of biliary cholesterol, together with decreased gallbladder contraction. These changes are a consequence of increased levels of estrogen and progesterone during pregnancy, which normalize after birth; cholelithiasis, sometimes diagnosed during the late gestation period, has proven on occasion to resolve during the early postpartum period.

Overall genetic factors: Epidemiologic studies using ultrasonography or cholecystographic screening show a very dissimilar prevalence of gallstone disease among various populations and ethnic groups. The greatest prevalence of cholelithiasis has been found among some North American Indians, Chileans, and Mexican Americans. Gallbladder disease, including gallbladder cancer, has become endemic in Bolivia and Chile related in part to the presence of lithogenetic genes with a very high penetration in South America. The lowest prevalence of cholelithiasis has been observed among the Japanese.

Family history: The incidence of cholelithiasis is increased among patients with a family history of gallstones. In subjects in whom both parents have gallstones, the prevalence of cholelithiasis increased to 14% compared with 12% among those with one parent with gallstones, and 6% among those with no family history.

Diet: A diet high in fat and cholesterol may increase biliary secretion of cholesterol and cholesterol saturation of bile, whereas diets rich in non-saturated fat and fiber may be protective against cholelithiasis.

Hormone replacement treatment: Estrogen treatment in both humans and experimental animals increases incidence of cholelithiasis by altering the cholesterol saturation in bile.

Other factors: Cholelithiasis is also increased in type 2 diabetes mellitus, cystic fibrosis, some dyslipidemias, long-term total parenteral nutrition, prolonged fasting, and short bowel syndrome.

Pathogenesis of Gallstone Formation

Bile contains cholesterol, bile pigments (from broken-down hemoglobin), various biliary proteins, and phospholipids. If the relative concentration ratios of these vary, cholelithiasis may occur resulting in several types of stones.

Cholesterol stones are large, often solitary, and radiolucent. In contrast, *pigment stones* are black, small, friable, irregular, and radiolucent. In most cases, pigment stones form as a result of the metabolic products of hemoglobin, and thus develop commonly in hemolytic disease (e.g., sickle cell anemia, hereditary spherocytosis, thalassemia). *Mixed stones* are usually multiple, faceted (calcium salts, pigment, and cholesterol), and radiopaque. *Brown pigment stones* are soft, earthy, brown stones that tend to form in the common bile duct as a result of stasis and infection within the biliary tree; primary common bile duct stones are usually these brown pigment stones. Certain species of *Escherichia coli* and *Klebsiella* produce glucuronidase, which is believed to convert soluble conjugated bilirubin back to the insoluble unconjugated state, leading to the formation of these stones.

Among these different kinds of stones, cholesterol stones account for 80% of patients with cholelithiasis. The etiology of cholesterol gallstones is multifactorial, with interaction from genetic and environmental factors related to abnormalities in cholesterol metabolism and bile secretion. Biliary cholesterol is primarily from preformed lipoprotein cholesterol with only a minor contribution of cholesterol generated from endogenous hepatic synthesis. Irrespective of the source, cholesterol is sorted and transported within the hepatocyte to the canalicular region for biliary secretion. This complex and highly regulated trafficking of transhepatic cholesterol into the bile involves multiple genes controlling cholesterol transport, whose expression is regulated by the concerted activity of sterol-activated transcriptional factors. The understanding of the hepatic determinants of biliary cholesterol elimination is relevant for overall cholesterol homeostasis and diseases of gallstone formation.

Clinical Presentation

Most subjects with cholelithiasis are asymptomatic, and only about 1–2% of these patients will develop symptoms each year. In contrast, others with gallstones develop quite characteristic presentations. Physical signs or symptoms of cholelithiasis include the following.

Biliary colic: This characteristic type of presentation is the most common symptom and results from the gallbladder. Gallbladder distension and inability to empty occurs secondary to mechanical or even functional obstruction of the cystic duct by a gallstone present in the cystic duct and is exacerbated by secretion of cholecystokinin, which stimulates gallbladder contraction. Biliary colic may also arise from a stone acutely or intermittently obstructing the extrahepatic biliary tree with acute distension of the bile duct and/or gallbladder.

The typical pain of biliary "colic" has a *slow* crescendo/decrescendo onset/resolution that occurs almost exclusively in the evening or night time. The term "colic" is really a misnomer in that the characteristic of the pain is not a colic but rather a slow onset of increasing constant pain that lasts 1–3 h and then resolves slowly. Although it tends to occur 1–3 h after a meal, biliary colic is extremely unusual after breakfast and maybe less so after lunch, but it is much more common after the evening meal. Gallbladder pain is typically in the right upper abdomen but can radiate to the right shoulder or right scapular region posteriorly. True epigastric pain can occur from gallbladder, but epigastric pain should alert the clinician to the possibility of choledocholithiasis.

Another type of gallbladder pain occurs secondary to a chronically obstructed, non-functioning gallbladder. The pain related to this condition tends to be a persistent, aching right upper quadrant discomfort that is unrelated to meals.

Atypical abdominal symptoms: Non-specific abdominal pain, nausea, vomiting, a feeling of bloating, heartburn, and "intolerance" to fatty foods may be present among patients with cholelithiasis. These atypical symptoms are not specific for gallbladder disease and may have other causes; other abdominal pathologies should be evaluated and excluded before suggesting cholecystectomy based solely on these atypical symptoms.

Jaundice: The presence of jaundice associated with cholelithiasis suggests strongly the presence of obstruction of the bile duct and/or associated hepatic disease. Jaundice may occur as a progressive onset without fever or pain, but this type of clinical presentation should suggest the presence of a neoplastic process (gallbladder, biliary, pancreatic) causing a total biliary obstruction. In contrast, a more acute presentation of jaundice associated with fever, chills, abdominal pain, but non-progressive jaundice in the presence of gallstones should prompt consideration of choledocholithiasis, acute cholecystitis, acute pancreatitis, or hepatitis. An uncommon group is those with Mirizzi's syndrome in whom a cystic duct stone causes obstruction of the common bile duct in the region of entry of the cystic duct into the choledochus.

Palpable gallbladder: Abdominal palpation of the gallbladder may be possible with either acute or chronic distension of the gallbladder. Severe tenderness on palpation of a distended gallbladder is highly suggestive of acute cholecystitis. Other findings on physical examination may include mild to moderate abdominal distension and tenderness to palpation in the right upper quadrant with inspiration as the gallbladder descends (Murphy's sign) and/or epigastrium. The absence of muscle rigidity or rebound tenderness suggests chronic cystic duct obstruction and not acute cholecystitis.

Diagnosis

Laboratory evaluation: A mild leukocytosis may be evident with symptomatic cholelithiasis; however, higher WBC counts (>12,000) suggest the presence of acute cholecystitis or associated complications. Hepatic function tests, such as serum bilirubin concentration and alkaline phosphatase and aspartate transaminase activity, may also be helpful in evaluation of a patient with cholelithiasis. When the levels of these liver function tests are increased, acute cholecystitis or choledocholithiasis should be suspected. Increases in serum amylase or lipase activity may suggest the presence of choledocholithiasis with associated acute pancreatitis.

Imaging studies: In patients with suspected cholelithiasis, ultrasonography provides the most effective, inexpensive, noninvasive initial imaging method. Ultrasonography (US) has a 95% sensitivity and 97% positive predictive value (PPV) for cholelithiasis. In most patients with cholelithiasis, gallstones are radiolucent, and although not evident on an abdominal radiograph, they still have a characteristic posterior, ecogenic shadow.

In addition to documenting the presence of gallstones, US can also assess gallbladder wall thickening or calcification, intrahepatic and/or extrahepatic duct dilation, and pericholecystic fluid, and may also assess surrounding organs and structures. A gallbladder wall thickness greater than 3 mm is considered abnormal. When the wall is >3 mm and there is associated pericholecystic fluid, gallbladder distension, impacted stone, or abdominal tenderness during the US examination, acute cholecystitis should be suspected.

US also allows evaluation of the intra and extrahepatic biliary system. Common bile duct (CBD) dilation >7 mm on US suggests choledocholithiasis, although the obstructive stone(s) may not be observed. The CBD is often difficult to visualize due to overlying intestinal gas from the colon or duodenum precluding accurate assessment. Overall sensitivity of US in identifying choledocholithiasis is only about 50%.

MR cholangio-pancreatography (MRCP) and abdominal CT are useful complementary studies after US, especially when associated choledocholithiasis or neoplasia is suspected. Abdominal CT has a limited sensitivity for the diagnosis of cholelithiasis and choledocholithiasis, although CT is extremely useful in patients with a suspected gallbladder neoplasm, because it will help to confirm the diagnosis, presence or absence of liver extension, dilation of the biliary tree, and the presence of lymph node metastases.

MRCP also has good diagnostic value for small neoplasms and especially choledocholithiasis with an 89–96% sensitivity

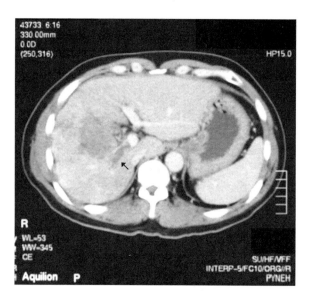

FIGURE 9.4. CT of a patient with HCC. The right portal vein was invaded by direct extension of the tumor (arrow).

Presentation

HCC usually grows silently until it reaches a large size and causes symptoms of compression on adjacent viscera. Thus, the majority of patients with resectable HCC do not have symptoms. Most of the resectable tumors are detected on screening. Nevertheless, some patients do have an early symptom of distending discomfort which could be due to rapid tumor growth. Sudden epigastric pain may be due to intratumoral bleeding leading to distension of the liver capsule. Continuous intratumoral bleeding will lead to rupture of HCC (and hence shock and peritonitis), especially when it is superficial. Hemoperitoneum and spillage of cancer cells into the peritoneal cavity account for poor short-and long-term survival; however, a minor degree of hemoperitoneum may be found at laparotomy and is due to splitting of the liver overlying the rapidly expanding HCC rather than actual rupture of HCC. In such a situation, abdominal pain is less severe, hemodynamic disturbance is less obvious, liver function is less impaired, and the prognosis is not necessarily worsened.

In other cases, the presenting symptom is abdominal distension, possibly due to huge hepatomegaly or ascites. Sometimes, the patients present with hemoptysis, bone pain, or pathologic fracture. HCC may also produce a hormone-like substance and a para-neoplastic syndrome such as diarrhea, hypercalcemia, or polycythemia. Jaundice may be the first presentation (Fig. 9.5) and may be due to compression or infiltration of the common hepatic duct by a large hilar HCC or tumor fragment dislodged from the intrahepatic duct into the common bile duct. In the latter situation, the patient may also present with acute cholangitis or pancreatitis.

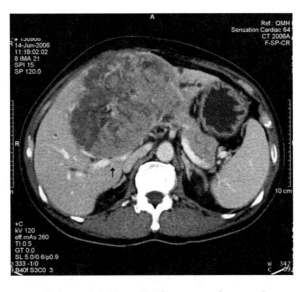

FIGURE 9.5. A large left liver HCC compressing on the common hepatic duct and portal vein (arrow). The patient presented with painless obstructive jaundice. At laparotomy, evidence of portal hypertension was also noted.

Imaging/Diagnosis

The routine x-ray offers no role in diagnosis except in advanced stages when the right diaphragm is elevated. The majority of small HCC(<2 cm) are detected by ultrasonographic screening of patients with cirrhosis or hepatitis B carriers. On ultrasonography, small HCC appear as a hypoechoic, isoechoic, or hyperechoic lesion, whereas larger HCC are usually heterogeneous in appearance. Contrast-enhanced ultrasonography can improve detection of isoechoic tumors and can differentiate them from other hepatic tumors. The enhancement pattern is similar to that of computed tomography (CT) or magnetic resonance imaging (MRI).

Contrast-enhanced CT and MRI are important diagnostic modalities in the recognition and staging of HCC. Contrast-enhancement in the arterial phase (about 30 s after contrast administration) and rapid washout in the portovenous phase (about 90 seconds after contrast administration) is the typical pattern of HCC. In addition, the topographic relationship of the tumor with major portal pedicles and hepatic veins is delineated clearly for planning of treatment. Hepatic angiography and porto-venography are performed rarely nowadays, because CT or MRI provides equally accurate assessment. Extrahepatic spread can also be delineated on CT or MRI. In case of doubt about the diagnosis and extent of spread, PET scans can be helpful, but both (18)F-FDG and ^{11}C-acetate should be used in the examination, because well-differentiated HCC are detected by ^{11}C-acetate radio-tracer, but not by (18) F-FDG; PET scan may replace bone scan in the evaluation of a patient with HCC for liver transplantation.

Serology Diagnosis

Serum alpha feto-protein (AFP) is a well-established tumor marker used in the diagnosis of HCC. The serum level of AFP, said to be diagnostic for HCC, varies from center to center; however, a diagnostic level is meaningless, because the amount of AFP produced by the tumors varies widely and is not proportional to tumor size. About 20–40% of HCC, even when large, may not produce sufficient amounts of AFP to be detectable in blood. Perhaps a rising trend, even within the normal reference range, is an indication of a growing tumor. Falsely high AFP levels may be found in patients with hepatitis B virus reactivation or ongoing hepatitis C infection. Such a phenomenon must be borne in mind when interpreting the serum AFP level in a patient with HCC.

In Japan, AFP-L3 and des-gamma-carboxyprothrombin (a protein induced by vitamin K antagonist II, PIVKA-II) are also used widely for diagnosis of HCC. A number of other novel markers have also been developed to cover the deficiency of AFP. None has been established for routine use yet.

Tumor Biopsy

Cytologic or histologic confirmation of HCC is needed when the lesion is inoperable and when the imaging is inconclusive of HCC. Tumor biopsy is also needed when the serum AFP is not increased and when conservative or non-operative treatment is planned. Tumor biopsy, however, is not without risk. Hemoperitoneum, arteriovenous fistula, and hemobilia are serious potential complications of tumor biopsy and may cause hepatic decompensation and death. Tumor seeding into the peritoneal cavity or along the needle track may be seen if the patient survives long enough. In the presence of ascites, tumor biopsy is contraindicated. Therefore, the European Association of Study of the Liver suggested that tumor biopsy is not needed if two coincident imaging techniques have shown typical arterial hyper-vascularization or when arterial enhancement is seen in one imaging technique together with increased serum AFP > 400 ng/ml.

Apart from tumor biopsy, liver biopsy of the contralateral liver is also advocated for assessment of the extent of hepatic fibrosis, which may have prognostic value. Again, the procedure is invasive. A non-invasive ultrasonography (Fibroscan) has been developed for assessment of liver fibrosis and may provide useful information in the future.

Treatment

Both partial hepatectomy and liver transplantation are the effective treatments. Other treatments available currently include transarterial chemoembolization (TACE), radiofrequency ablation, and percutaneous alcohol or acetic acid injection.

Before a treatment plan is offered, multiple aspects of the following assessment must be made.

Tumor Status

The size and number of tumor nodules may be recognized by ultrasonography, CT, MRI, or PET scan.The proximity of the tumor to a major vascular pedicle and possible invasion is a concern for planning partial hepatectomy or radiofrequency ablation. Tumor invasion into the inferior vena cava or portal vein is a definite contraindication for operative exploration, but isolated portal vein thrombosis can be secondary to cirrhosis and portal hypertension. In the latter situation, liver transplantation is still possible. Ascites may be due to cirrhosis, but peritoneal spread may account for small amounts of fluid near the tumor. Blood clot adjacent to the tumor can be recognized by CT and is an indication of recent rupture and possible peritoneal spread. The sites of regional lymph node spread include the hepato-duodenal ligament, suprahepatic-subdiaphragmatic region, and behind the head of the pancreas. CT of the thorax or PET scan using dual radio-tracers is recommended for large HCC and those with hepatic vein invasion.

Liver Function Status

Assessment of liver function is mandatory to determine whether the patient can tolerate the proposed treatment. For partial hepatectomy, assessment of liver function is of paramount importance, because part of the uninvolved liver is removed with the tumor. For radiofrequency ablation, though a small part of the liver surrounding the tumor is ablated and little functional loss is anticipated, the systemic inflammatory response is sometimes excessive, and the patient may succumb to liver failure if the liver function is suboptimal. For TACE, the non-tumorous liver may also be affected by the treatment, and post-TACE liver failure may occur.

Liver function may be assessed by clinical examination. Presence of ascites, jaundice, and hepatic encephalopathy indicates that any treatment except liver transplantation is inappropriate. Laboratory assessment includes a platelet count, international normalized ratio (prothrombin time), and serum bilirubin and albumin levels. The Child-Pugh classification of liver function is a useful guide for partial hepatectomy, but it is important to note that two of the five parameters (ascites and encephalopathy) are not quantitative. In general, patients with Child-Pugh class A liver function are suitable candidates for partial hepatectomy. Child-Pugh B patients are borderline cases for local resection of a peripherally situated tumor. Child-Pugh C patients are definitely not candidates for partial hepatectomy. For other local treatments, Child-Pugh A and B patients may have low complication rates after the procedures, whereas Child-Pugh C patients represent a high risk; however, no detailed study has been carried out to date on the tolerance of cirrhotic patients to radiofrequency ablation and TACE.

Among Child-Pugh A patients, the actual liver function varies, and operative mortality may be as high as 13% after major hepatectomy. A better quantitative test of risk of postoperative liver failure is the indocyanine green (ICG) clearance test. The normal value is 10% retention at 15 min after intravenous administration of ICG. Major hepatectomy is still feasible if the ICG retention rate at 15 min is 14%. If blood loss is not excessive and blood transfusion not required, patients with 18% retention at 15 min may survive major hepatectomy.

Remnant Liver Volume Status

The survival of patients after partial hepatectomy or radiofrequency ablation depends upon the function and volume of the remnant liver. A remnant liver volume >30% is sufficient for postoperative survival; however, for patients with chronic liver disease, remnant liver volume >40% is needed. When the estimated remnant liver would be insufficient and the non-tumorous liver to be resected with the liver neoplasm is large in volume, portal vein embolization can be performed to induce liver atrophy of the resected side and hypertrophy of the remnant side. This procedure, however, is not applicable to patients with moderate or severe cirrhosis.

General Status

The purpose of assessment is to determine whether the patient has concomitant medical disease that makes the treatment dangerous. Patients with serious medical disease, e.g. recent myocardial infarction, stroke, uremia and severe chronic obstructive airwaydisease, are not candidates for partial hepatectomy or radiofrequency ablation via laparotomy. Presently, with better selection of patients, the operative mortality rate has been reduced markedly(<3%), but the complication rate remains high. Concomitant medical disease is the most important contributory factor to the high complication rate.

Partial Hepatectomy

Right or left hepatectomy is indicated when the tumor is confined to one side of the liver, when the remnant liver volume is sufficient, and when the liver function is optimal. For small tumors(<2 cm), the ideal treatment would be resection of the liver segment harboring the tumor together with the adjacent segments to eradicate possible spread from portal vein branches. It is also necessary to preserve non-tumorous liver. Currently, the principle of resection consists of removal of the tumor with a tumor-free margin of at least 5mm, little blood loss, no blood transfusion, maximal preservation of non-tumorous liver, and preferably minimum manipulation of primary neoplasm (Fig. 9.6). To reduce blood loss, intermittent inflow vascular occlusion can be employed, but the accumulated occlusion time should not exceed 120 min. Many hepatic surgeons believe that the best liver transection device is the ultrasonic dissector, despite its slowness. Other devices, e.g. harmonic scalpel, Tissue-Link, and others that deliver energy to coagulate the liver parenchyma, tend to induce liver necrosis and fail to identify clearly the intrahepatic portal pedicles and hepatic vein, which serve as important land-marks for safe and complete resection of hemiliver or liver segment.

The extent of hepatectomy is classified as major or minor, but there is no rigid rule of extent of hepatectomy. For example, a right hepatectomy can be carried out together with resection of a superficial tumor nodule in the left liver; the caudate lobe resection is included in a right hepatectomy. Segment V, VI, VII resection is performed to preserve segment VIII for a relatively small liver. Avoidance of blood loss and protection of the liver remnant from ischemic injury are the two important strategies to ensure postoperative survival. Meticulous attention to avoid bile leakage and bile duct injury is mandatory for success. In the latter situation, operative cholangiography is the prerequisite investigation.

Currently, partial hepatectomy for HCC can be performed with nearly 0% hospital mortality, about 30% complication rate, a 5-year survival of 49%, and a 10-year survival of 30%. Better survival rates are obtained for patients with TNM stages I and II (5-year survival of 80% and 60%, respectively).

Liver Transplantation

A remarkable advance has been the use of liver transplantation for selected patients with HCC arising in a cirrhotic liver. Liver transplantation is indicated for patients with Child-Pugh

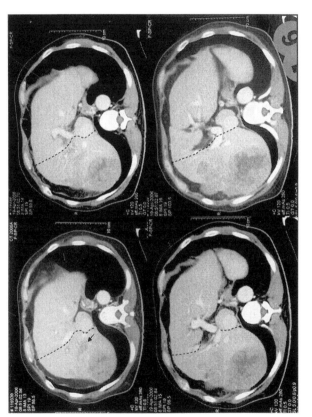

FIGURE 9.6. CT of a patient with right liver HCC. The arrow indicates the right hepatic vein invaded by HCC. Fluid collection outside the liver was also noted. The dotted line represents the line of liver transection. The operation was performed by the anterior approach, i.e. the liver transection was done without prior right liver mobilization to avoid dissemination of cancer cells into the systemic circulation.

class B or C liver function and those without concomitant major medical diseases. Patients should be selected carefully based on formal radiologic criteria. Patients with solitary neoplasms <5 cm or those with ≤3 tumors, each of which is ≤3 cm, are favorable candidates; this subset of patients has a 5-year survival of about 75–80%. Slight extension of the aforementioned criteria has been advocated recently to allow more patients to benefit from liver transplantation without jeopardizing the long-term survival rate. In contrast, use of liver transplantation for larger HCC or those with multiple satellite lesions is not indicated, because the survival is not better than after resective or ablative procedures. Nevertheless, whatever the selection criteria based on imaging, up to 25% of the patients have HCC recurrence after liver transplantation. The deficiency is that the size and number of tumor nodules do not reflect the actual pathologic features or biologic behavior. Well-differentiated HCC and those without vascular invasion have excellent prognosis after liver transplantation, but histologic information would not be available unless liver biopsy is performed or the explant is available. Recent research aims at identification of biologic markers of aggressiveness in patients' pre-transplant blood specimen that can predict post-transplant recurrence.

TACE

In this treatment of transarterial chemoembolization, a mixture of Lipiodol and a chemotherapeutic agent is administered into the artery feeding the HCC, followed by embolization and occlusion of the artery. Lipiodol has affinity for HCC and carries with it the chemotherapeutic agent in high local concentration directly to the HCC. Mixing of Lipiodol with the chemotherapeutic agent is by the syringe-pump method. Various combinations of chemotherapeutic agents have been advocated, but cisplatin appears to form a mixture with Lipiodol that is stable for 1–2 hours, which is more stable than the other chemotherapeutic agents. After injecting this mixture into the hepatic artery, the terminal branches of the feeding artery will be occluded, causing ischemia. Later, the chemotherapeutic agent will be released to act on the tumor. Subsequent embolization of the feeding artery is useful to prevent flushing away of the mixture by blood flow, but recent practice tends to omit the subsequent embolization, because the result appears to be equally satisfactory for small HCC without embolization and potentially harmful effects to the liver can be avoided.

TACE not only prolongs survival of patients with inoperable HCC, but it has also been used as a "bridge" or a means to "down-stage" the tumor to deceased donor liver transplantation. TACE is not effective against large HCC, however, and recurrence, especially at the periphery of the tumor, is frequent. The high recurrence rate may be due to stimulation of angiogenesis. Thus, an anti-angiogenesis treatment may be considered with TACE.

TACE is not without risk. Liver failure, liver abscess, and biloma are potentially lethal complications. Patients with Child-Pugh class C liver function tolerate TACE poorly. Thus, its role as a bridge to liver transplantation is applicable only in patients with Child-Pugh A and B cirrhosis. Overall, the 5-year survival rate of patients treated by TACE alone is about 20%.

Radiofrequency Ablation

This, non-resective treatment consists of insertion of an electrode into the tumor either percutaneously or transhepatically at the time of operation under CT or ultrasonography guidance; local heat is generated within the tumor during the subsequent delivery of energy via the electrode. The local temperature reaches 60°C, coagulating the tumor. RFA is most suitable for tumors ≤3–5 cm. Larger tumors can be treated by RFA, but preferably in several sessions to avoid excessive systemic inflammatory response. Percutaneous RFA, however, is not suitable for lesions near the bowel, diaphragm, and liver hilum. For these situation, an open approach is preferred, with the bowel or diaphragm packed away from the tumor before application of radiofrequency. For lesions close to the liver hilum, cold saline flushing of the common bile duct via cystic duct cannulation will decrease the injury to the hepatic duct. The reported mortality rate from RFA is low(<1%), but serious complications may occur, including liver abscess, hepatic duct damage leading to biloma, bowel perforation, gallbladder necrosis, hemoglobinuria, renal failure, and liver failure.

Overall, the 5-year survival of patients treated by RFA alone is about 33%. There has been an increasing tendency in recent years to treat potentially resectable HCC ($\leq$ 5 cm) by RFA. A randomized trial suggests that RFA for small HCC is as effective as formal operative resection.

Intralesional Alcohol Ablation

This treatment consists of injection of 95% alcohol into the tumor by percutaneous needle puncture under ultrasonography guidance. The mode of action is by drawing water from the cells leading to desiccation of the tumor. Although this approach is applicable to small tumors (<3 cm), the alcohol is less able to penetrate the tumor capsule, and therefore, may not finally treat the cancer cells that have invaded across the tumor capsule. Acetic acid is able to penetrate the tumor capsule and has been used to replace alcohol; however, the pattern of spread of alcohol and acetic acid across the lesion is unpredictable. Both treatments have been essentially replaced by RFA in recent years.

Other Treatments

Because the current treatments are not entirely effective and their applications are limited, new treatments are being developed. Recently investigated modalities include local radioisotope therapy (Yttrium 90, Iodine 131), Tomo Therapy, and High Intensity Focused Ultrasound. The latter two modalities have the advantage of being totally non-invasive, but data are not yet sufficient to recommend them as routine procedures.

Choice of Treatment

Choosing the appropriate treatment for individual patients depends on the medical condition of the patient, size and location of the lesion(s), liver function, volume of the remnant liver, and availability of local expertise. Occasionally, the tumor can be downstaged by local or systemic chemotherapy and become resectable. Thus, young patients with good liver function free of concomitant medical disease should be offered aggressive treatment. Whatever the initial treatment, recurrence of HCC is common, and apart from liver transplantation, the incidence is as high as 60% in the first year. Combination of the aforementioned treatment modalities or their sequential use for recurrent HCC that developed during the course of the disease is the logical approach. For example, partial hepatectomy may be the first treatment. Subsequent recurrences can be treated by RFA, TACE, or even liver transplantation. The overall survival rate is improved if early recurrence is detected by careful surveillance and treated aggressively and promptly by the same or different modality.

Screening

Since the prognosis of HCC treatment depends on the tumor size and early HCC are asymptomatic, recent efforts to improve the overall outcome have targeted screening of the population at risk for development of HCC. The screened subjects are those with cirrhosis, hepatitis B or C carriers, and family members of HCC who are screened by ultrasonography and serum AFP measurement simultaneously at

6-to 12-month intervals. Both ultrasonography and AFP measurement are performed to compensate for deficiencies of each. The average size of HCC detected by such mode of surveillance is about 2 cm. Theoretically and ideally, about 90% of HCC can be detected by such screening. In practice, however, many early HCC are missed by this combination, especially in cirrhotic patients. More cost-effective surveillance methods are needed.

Prevention

Nationwide hepatitis B vaccination of children reduces the incidence of HCC among the population at risk. Treatment of hepatitis B by lamivudine and hepatitis C by interferon is beneficial in reducing the development of HCC among these patients. Recently, patients with HCC have been treated with lamivudine or interferon after the initial radical treatment, hoping to reduce the incidence of recurrence. The efficacy has not been confirmed yet, but this approach seems logical.

Selected Readings

Bruix J, Sherman M, Llovet JM, et al. (2001) Clinical management of hepatocellular carcinoma. Conclusions of the Barcelona-2000 EASL conference. European Association for the Study of the Liver. J Hepatol 35:421–430

Chen MS, Li JQ, Zheng Y, et al. (2006) A prospective randomized trial comparing percutaneous local ablative therapy and partial hepatectomy for small hepatocellular carcinoma. Ann Surg 243:321–328

Chien YC, Jan CF, Kuo HS, et al. (2006) Nationwide hepatitis B vaccination program in Taiwan: effectiveness in the 20 years after it was launched. Epidemiol Rev Jun [Epub ahead of print]

Lam CM, Fan ST, Lo CM, et al. (1999) Major hepatectomy for hepatocellular carcinoma in patients with an unsatisfactory indocyanine green clearance test. Br J Surg 86:1012–1017

Lau WY, Ho SK, Yu SC, et al. (2004) Salvage surgery following downstaging of unresectable hepatocellular carcinoma. Ann Surg 240:299–305

Poon RTP, Fan ST, Lo CM, et al. (2002) Long-term survival and pattern of recurrence after resection of small hepatocellular carcinoma in patients with preserved liver function: implications for a strategy of salvage transplantation. Ann Surg 235:373–382

Yang ZF, Poon RTP, To J, et al. (2004) The potential role of hypoxia inducible factor 1alpha in tumor progression after hypoxia and chemotherapy in hepatocellular carcinoma. Cancer Res 64:5496–5503

Zhu LX, Wang GS, Fan ST (1996) Spontaneous rupture of hepatocellular carcinoma. Br J Surg 83:602–607

10
Metastatic Cancer of the Liver

**Matteo Donadon, Gareth Morris-Stiff,
and Jean-Nicolas Vauthey**

Pearls and Pitfalls

- If untreated, patients with colorectal liver metastases have an overall 5-year survival <5%, with a median survival of 12–15 months.
- Selected patients with colorectal liver metastases are candidates for curative hepatic resection with 5-year survival approaching 60%.
- Perioperative mortality and morbidity rates are <5% and 40%, respectively.
- Absolute contraindications for resection are peritoneal carcinomatosis, multiple extrahepatic sites of metastatic disease, and inability to achieve an R0 resection.
- Multiple but resectable hepatic metastases are not necessarily a contraindication to resection.
- Resectable lung metastases are also not necessarily a contraindication to resection.
- At present, the role of interstitial therapy should be confined to unresectable lesions
- Serum CEA levels are increased in 75% of patients with liver metastases and serve as markers of disease.

K.I. Bland et al. (eds.), *Liver and Biliary Surgery*,
DOI 10.1007/978-1-84996-429-6_10,
© Springer-Verlag London Limited 2011

- Preoperative chemotherapy and portal vein embolization (PVE) are beneficial in potentially downsizing lesions in patients with initially unresectable disease to allow curative resection.
- Liver resection for hepatic metastases from neuroendocrine cancer and possibly breast cancer has a role, but no good data support resection of other metastatic neoplasms.
- Liver transplantation is generally not considered for unresectable hepatic metastases.
- Predictors of recurrence are R1 status, synchronous presentation of liver metastases with colon cancer, stage of colon cancer, size and number of metastases, preoperative CEA, and extrahepatic metastases.

Multidisciplinary Approach to Metastatic Cancer of the Liver

The liver is the most common site of metastases from a variety of primary cancers, particularly those originating from the gastrointestinal tract. In autopsy series of patients dying of neoplasia, hepatic metastases are found in up to 36% of patients, the most frequent primary sites being: colon and rectum, lung, pancreas, breast, and stomach. The prognosis of patients with untreated liver metastases is generally verypoor, and if untreated, the majorityof such patients succumb to their disease within 12 months of diagnosis.

The increase in diagnosis and recognition of the importance of close follow-up of gastrointestinal malignancies during the past decade has led to a corresponding increase in the identification of liver metastases. These lesions are now being detected at an earlier stage as a result of improvements in imaging techniques and an increased awareness of potential treatment options amongst the medical community. As a result, patients who until a few years ago were considered candidates only for palliative care are nowadays being offered a chance of cure, because of a multidisciplinary and multi-modality approach in which liver resection is the key.

Operative Resection of Colorectal Liver Metastases

Colorectal cancer is the second leading cause of cancer-related mortality worldwide, and every year more than 140,000 patients in the Unites States are diagnosed with this disease. Even though 85% of patients have neoplasms amenable to curative resection at the time of diagnosis, the disease recurs in more than half of the patients within 5 years. The most frequent sites of colorectal metastases are the liver, which accounts for 30–60% of colorectal metastases, and the lung, representing 20–30%. Up to 25% of patients have liver metastases detected at the time of diagnosis of the primary colorectal neoplasm (synchronous metastases), while the remaining 30% develop liver metastases after their initial diagnosis (metachronous metastases). Without treatment, the median survival of patients with colorectal liver metastases is 12–15 months, and the 5-year survival rate is less than 5%. Many treatment modalities have been investigated to prolong the survival of patients with colorectal liver metastases, but liver resection remains the only method associated with long-term survival.

Natural History of Untreated Colorectal Liver Metastases

The natural history of untreated colorectal liver metastases has been defined clearly by studies that examined the impact of operative treatment on survival in the era predating the use of systemic chemotherapy. Scheele et al. reviewed 1,209 patients with colorectal liver metastases and compared three subgroups of patients: 921 who underwent a debulking procedure, hepatic arterial infusion, or palliative care; 62 who were untreated; and 226 patients who underwent curative resection. Only the curative resection group had 5-year survivors with 5-and 10-year survival rates in this cohort of 40% and 27%, respectively. In another study, Scheele et al. (1995) showed that patients who underwent curative resection and were cancer-free at 5 years, had an 88% probability of being cancer-free at 10 years. This study provides the best presumptive evidence that operative resection for colorectal liver metastases can modify directly the natural history of disease and improve long-term survival.

Indications and Contraindications to Operative Resection

Traditionally, contraindications to resection of colorectal liver metastases have been unresectable liver disease and extrahepatic disease (Table 10.1). In many studies, multiple hepatic metastases and the presence of bilobar disease were said to be associated with a worse prognosis, especially in patients with more than four hepatic metastases, because there was said to be a high risk of recurrence after operative resection. It is now recommended that patients with more than four hepatic metastases should undergo a thorough preoperative staging, and in this subset of patients, preoperative systemic chemotherapy should be considered, even if the disease is initially resectable. As such, the presence of multiple hepatic metastases is no longer considered an absolute contraindication to resection.

Another controversial area is the appropriateness of operative resection in patients with metastases in perihepatic lymph nodes, as their presence predicts a poor outcome after operation. Jaeck et al. showed recently that metastases in

TABLE 10.1. Contraindications to resection of colorectal liver metastases.

Relative	Absolute
Extrahepatic metastases	Peritoneal carcinomatosis
Colonic recurrence	Multiple extrahepatic metastases
Solitary resectable peritoneal metastasis	Inability to perform hepatic R0 resection
Hilar lymph nodes metastases	

hilar and perihepatic lymph nodes have a worse impact on prognosis than multiple liver metastases, increase in serum carcinoembryonic antigen (CEA) level, or even solitary resectable peritoneal disease. Therefore there is currently no indication for routine resection of perihepatic lymph nodes in patients with colorectal liver metastases.

Several authors have reported long-term survival in patients with resectable extrahepatic metas-tases. Elias et al. showed a 5-year overall survival rate of 28% in patients with more than five hepatic metastases and multiple sites of extrahepatic disease. Other studies have shown that long-term survival can be expected after complete resection (R0 resection) of colorectal metastases to the lung, even when these metastases are present at the time of diagnosis of the primary colorectal tumor.

Diagnosis and Preoperative Work-Up

Patients with primary colorectal cancer should undergo follow-up examinations, which differ in intensity and in the imaging modalities used according to the preference of the treating physician. Most follow-up protocols consist of physical examination, colonoscopy, measurement of serum levels of CEA and CA 19-9, and abdominal computed tomography (CT). CEA maybe of importance because the vast majority of patients with colorectal disease have an increase in serum CEA. After a curative colonic resection, levels fall to normal, and thus a secondary increase in serum CEA is indicative of recurrent or metastatic disease acting as a stimulus for radiologic localization. Increased serum levels of CEA are seen in greater than 75% of patients with colorectal liver metastases. Moreover, CEA represents one of the most important prognostic factors for long-term survival after resection of colorectal liver metastases. Recently, Adam et al. identified CA 19-9 as an important indicator of prognosis in patients undergoing hepatic resection; however, further confirmatory studies are necessary to support this finding prior to widespread implementation.

The preferred imaging modality for detection of colorectal liver metastases is CT, because it is available widely and allows simultaneous imaging of the thorax, liver, abdomen, and pelvis. We favor quadruple-phase (precontrast, arterial, portal, and delayed), multislice CT with rapid intravenous contrast injection (3–5 ml/s) and 2–5 mm cuts of the liver.

Fluorodeoxyglucose positron emission tomography (FDG-PET) has been used recently in the preoperative work-up of patients with colorectal liver metastases and has a role in selection of the best candidates for liver resection. A recent meta-analysis provided evidence that FDG-PET has greater sensitivity in the detection of colorectal liver metastases (95%) than helical CT (65%) or 1.5 T magnetic resonance imaging (MRI) (76%). The resolution of FDG-PET, however, remains inferior to that of CT or MRI, as does its specificity, especially in patients who have undergone preoperative chemotherapy; interpretation of results in this setting may be misleading.

Recently, the role of contrast-enhanced ultrasonography in the detection of colorectal metastases has been investigated. This new technique is promising, because it combines the well-established sensitivity of ultrasonography with the specificity of contrast examination, allowing further characterization of hepatic lesions. Furthermore, contrast-enhanced ultrasonography can be performed during intraoperative ultrasonography, now performed routinely during liver surgery, to give the surgeon an additional diagnostic tool in their diagnostic armamentarium.

Several groups have reported benefit from the use of intraoperative staging laparoscopy to minimize non-curative or "open and close" laparotomy rates which vary between 10% and 40%. This wide range probably reflects differences in the quality of the preoperative imaging work-up and also center-to-center variation in case-mix. Currently, we advocate laparoscopy in patients with advanced metastatic in whom hepatic injury from preoperative systemic chemotherapy is suspected.

Once patients have been diagnosed and a multidisciplinary decision is made that resection is appropriate, it is essential to ensure that they undergo repeat high quality imaging studies, with abdominal and pelvic CT (or MRI) within a month of the date of operation. A full cardiac and pulmonary work-up should be performed if past history and symptoms warrant. Baseline evaluation of hepatic function is mandatory before any hepatic resection to exclude dysfunction as a result of concomitant liver disease or side effects related to chemotherapy, because impaired hepatic function will have a negative impact in terms of a higher complication rate and may also limit the extent of the resection possible. In addition, candidates for extended resection, i.e., the removal of more than four adjacent segments, should undergo estimation of the future liver remnant (FLR) volume performed using CT volumetry of the liver.

Techniques for Resection

The current operative technique for liver resection is based on the segmental hepatic anatomy described by Couinaud in 1957. The surgical nomenclature used for anatomic resection is presented in Fig. 10.1. Non-anatomic resection, often referred to as atypical, wedge, or limited resection, consists of the removal of a part of the liver parenchyma without following the distribution of the portal vein branch that supplies the part of the liver being resected. Although some authors report a survival benefit for patients undergoing anatomic versus non-anatomic resection, no definitive evidence supports anatomic resection; long-term survival without local recurrence can be also achieved with nonanatomic resection even with minimal resection margins. Indeed, a recent multicenter analysis showed that the width of the negative surgical margin does not correlate with the probability of intrahepatic recurrence, only that the presence of a positive (versus negative) resection margin correlates with increased risk of intrahepatic recurrence.

Resection of hepatic colorectal metastases usually begins with a J-shaped incision in the right upper quadrant. After a

Extended right hepatectomy
or right trisectionectomy

Right hepatectomy   Bisegmentectomy II + III
or right hemihepatectomy   or left lateral sectionectomy

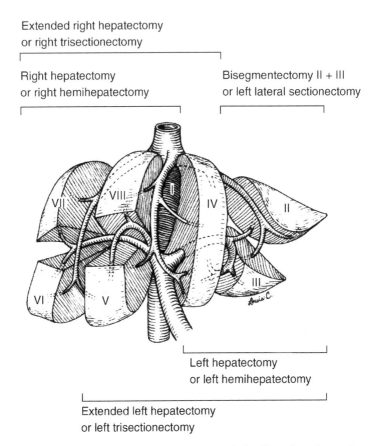

Left hepatectomy
or left hemihepatectomy

Extended left hepatectomy
or left trisectionectomy

FIGURE 10.1. Anatomic nomenclature of the liver based on the Brisbane 2000 hepatic resection nomenclature (Reprinted from Abdalla et al., 2004. With permission from Elsevier).

full exploration of the peritoneal cavity, the liver is mobilized by dividing all the relevant supporting ligaments. The liver is inspected, palpated, and evaluated further by intraoperative ultrasonography. Transection of the liver parenchyma can be carried out with one or more of a number of different current instruments, including ultrasonic dissectors and radiofrequency coagulators (Fig. 10.2), or with the more traditional

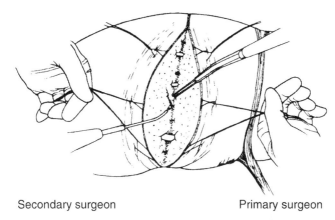

Secondary surgeon   Primary surgeon

FIGURE 10.2. Two-surgeon technique for hepatic parenchymal transection. The primary surgeon directs dissection with the ultrasonic dissector from the patient's left side and the secondary surgeon operates with the saline-linked cautery device from the patient's right side (Reprinted from Aloia et al., 2005. With permission from Lippincott, Williams & Wilkins).

crushing clamp technique. Generally, the resection is performed with control of the inflow (Pringle's maneuver) and sometimes of the outflow as well to reduce blood loss.

Perioperative Results

Liver resection is a well-established procedure that can be performed with mortality rates of less than 5%, with large centers now quoting rates of 1–2% and morbidity rates of less than 40%. The most powerful determinants of poor outcome after liver resection are preoperative cirrhosis or severe hepatic dysfunction, intraoperative bleeding, requirement for perioperative blood transfusions, insufficient remnant liver, and the development of postoperative infections. Indeed, these conditions can lead to hepatic failure, which although it occurs in fewer than 5% of patients, can have devastating consequences. Optimal patient selection, meticulous intraoperative technique, and careful postoperative management are essential to minimize surgical complications.

Long-Term Survival

Table 10.2 reports the main predictors of recurrence in major series of liver resection for colorectal metastases. Despite expanding indications for resection of colorectal metastases, overall 5-year survival is now reported to be as high as 58% in single and multi-institutional studies. The factors with the greatest influence on survival are margin status, stage of the primary colon neoplasm, preoperative plasma CEA level, size and number of hepatic lesions, and presence or absence of extrahepatic disease.

Surgical margin status is an important factor that influences long-term survival. Historically, a margin less than 1 cm was considered suboptimal, and some have even suggested that an anticipated margin less than 1 cm was a contraindication to resection. A recent study by Pawlik et al., however, showed that the width of resected margin (1–10 mm) did not affect local recurrence or survival, and indeed only the presence of a positive surgical margin (R1) was associated with an increased risk of recurrence (11%) and decreased survival (Fig. 10.3). Thus, patients with an anticipated surgical margin <1cm based on preoperative imaging or intraoperative findings could still undergo resection as long as negative margin is achievable.

Specific molecular markers have been linked with clinical outcome. In a recent study, our group demonstrated that human telomerase reverse transcriptase (hTERT) expression was associated independently with a worse prognosis after curative resection of colorectal liver metastases. In this study, hTERT-positive patients had a twofold increase in risk of death compared to hTERT-negative patients. This finding is important, because the use of molecular markers may prove useful to select high-risk patients who may benefit from preoperative systemic chemotherapy.

TABLE 10.2. Predictors of recurrence and long-term survival after resection for colorectal liver metastases.

Author, year	R1 status	Synchronous presentation	Primary nodes+	Size of meta stases	Number of meta stases	Preoperative CEA	Extrahepatic disease	5-Year survival
Gayowski, 1994	+	+	+	–	+	–	+	32%
Scheele, 1995	+	+	+	+	–	–	–	40%
Nordinger, 1996	+	+	+	+	+	+		28%
Jaeck, 1997	+	+	+	+	+	+	–	26%
Jamison, 1997	–			–	–			32%
Jenkins, 1997	+			–	–		+	25%
Elias, 1998	+	+	–	–	–	–	–	28%
Ambiru, 1999	+	–	+		+	+		23%
Fong, 1999	+		+		+	+	+	46%
Minagawa, 2000	–		–	–	+	–	–	38%
Figueras, 2001	+	–			+	+	+	53%
Choti, 2002	+	–	–	–	+	+		58%
Fernandez, 2004	+	–	–	–	+	–		58%
Abdalla, 2004	+	–		+	+			58%
Pawlik, 2005	+	–	–	+	+	+		58%

CEA, Carcino-Embryonic Antigen.

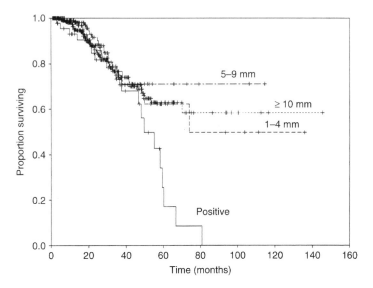

FIGURE 10.3. Survival after curative resection for colorectal liver metastases stratified by margin status. No difference in survival was seen in patients with negative surgical margins, regardless of the width of the margin (Reprinted from Pawlik et al., 2005. With permission from Lippincott, Williams & Wilkins).

Follow-Up

After resection of colorectal liver metastases, patients should be followed carefully to allow for early detection of recurrence. Follow-up evaluations after resection of colorectal liver metastases probably should include CEA and CA 19-9 measurements, liver function tests, pelvic and abdominal CT, and chest radiography every 3–6 months. A colonoscopy is also mandatory every 1–3 year after resection of the primary colonic resection. This schedule should be continued at least for 5 years after liver surgery.

Selected patients can undergo re-resection for recurrent colorectal liver metastases, and such patients can experience long-term survival. Adam et al. (2004) showed 5-year overall survival rates of 32% after the third hepatectomy, with no increase in postoperative morbidity or mortality rates.

Methods to Improve the Resectability of Colorectal Liver Metastases

Several strategies are available to render initially unresectable colorectal liver metastases resectable.

Neoadjuvant Systemic Chemotherapy

The development of new, more effective chemotherapy agents, such as oxaliplatin and irinotecan, has led to more widespread use of chemotherapy for patients with colorectal liver metastases – both those with resectable and those with unresectable disease at presentation. Indeed, both drugs, which are commonly used in combination with 5-fluorouracil-folinic acid-based regimens, can downsize liver metastases and control extrahepatic disease sites effectively. The use of these agents in conjunction with advances in techniques of parenchymal transection have led to a change in the concept of unresectable liver metastases and has expanded the population of patients who are potential candidates for hepatic resection.

The indications for neoadjuvant chemotherapy are based on risk factors for disease recurrence. Factors considered are size and number of metastases, disease-free interval between diagnosis of the primary colorectal neoplasm and the metastases, and presence of extrahepatic disease.

The more widespread use of neoadjuvant chemotherapy has given rise to a clinical dilemma: to prescribe or not to prescribe preoperative chemotherapy in patients with resectable colorectal liver metastases? This dilemma is not merely academic, because recent reports indicate an increase in the risk of adverse events after hepatic resection in patients treated preoperatively with systemic chemotherapy. Hepatocellular damage, including hepatic steatosis and more importantly steatohepatitis, has been described in patients treated preoperatively with irinotecan (yellow liver syndrome) and a sinusoidal obstruction syndrome is being described with increasing frequency in patients treated preoperatively with oxaliplatin (blue liver syndrome). These chemotherapy-related hepatic injuries can reduce the regenerative capacity of hepatocytes in response to major hepatectomy through alterations of nuclear factors such as nuclear factor-kappa B, which may interfere with the priming phase of liver regeneration. Therefore, the use of neoadjuvant chemotherapy should be considered cautiously in patients with resectable disease at presentation, in whom chemotherapy-related intrahepatic complications could necessitate modification of the surgical strategy or even prevent resection as a treatment option.

Portal Vein Embolization and Two-Stage Hepatectomy

Portal vein embolization (PVE) is used before major and extended hepatic resection to induce atrophy of the liver parenchyma to be resected (the embolized lobe) and compensatory hypertrophy of the liver to be preserved (the remnant liver), thereby increasing the hepatic reserve of the FLR. First developed in Japan, PVE is now frequently used by many centers worldwide and contributes to improved resectability rates for patients with liver cancer.

PVE is usually performed via a percutaneous, transhepatic approach consisting of ultrasound-guided puncture of a portal branch followed by embolization of the entire hemi-liver to be resected. Embolization can be achieved with a variety of substances, such as 100% ethanol, ethiodized oil, and cyanoacrylate, none are superior to the others. PVE is a well-established and well-tolerated procedure. The indications for PVE are based on the calculated FLR volume and the presence or absence of underlying liver disease. The FLR is calculated as the ratio of the FLR volume to the total liver volume (TLV)as calculated by CT, using a formula extrapolated from the association between

TLV and body surface area. This measurement allows for an estimation of the hepatic metabolic demand for each patient. The presence of underlying liver disease is another important factor to consider, because severely damaged livers may not have the capacity to regenerate. Both cirrhosis and severe steatosis have been found to impair liver regeneration after major hepatectomy. The use of PVE in these settings will allow hypertrophy of the remnant liver, albeit at a slower rate than for healthy liver, thus reducing the risk of subsequent hepatectomy.

Hypertrophy of the FLR after PVE is expected within the first month. The greatest increase in FLR occurs within the first 3 weeks, after which regeneration reaches a plateau. Hypertrophy of the nonembolized liver is regulated mainly by transforming growth factor-alpha, whose serum level has been reported as peaking at day20 after PVE and thereafter reaching a plateau. Thus, 3–4 weeks should be considered the optimum time interval to assess the hypertrophy response to PVE. In addition to the absolute volume of hypertrophy, the rate of hypertrophy is important, and we desire a 5% increase within the first month after PVE.

There is little agreement on the minimal FLR volume needed to avoid the small-for-size syndrome. The surgical series published to date report different methods of measurement of liver volume and include patients with considerably different degrees of underlying liver disease. A functional residual liver volume of <20% is associated with an increase in postoperative morbidity. In general, for patients with a normal underlying liver, resection is acceptable when the functional residual liver volume is >20%. In patients with injured liver, >30% is required, while in patients with cirrhosis or steatohepatitis, more than 40% is desired.

The role of PVE in permitting an R0 resection in patients with multiple bilobar disease has been investigated recently by Jaeck et al. who proposed the novel approach of two-stage hepatectomy, via removal of metastases in the left liver during first-stage hepatectomy and removal of metastases in the right liver during the second-stage. The second stage can be performed with or without preoperative PVE, depending on the functional residual liver volume. This approach should be considered in patients not eligible for R0 resection performed within the context of a single procedure.

Interstitial Therapies

Interstitial therapies for colorectal liver metastases have been in use for many years. Ethanol injection, cryosurgery, and microwave ablation have been utilized for local control of disease, generally with only short-term success. Currently, the most commonly used interstitial therapy is radiofrequency thermal ablation (RFA), which requires placement of an electrode within the liver tumor under radiologic guidance (ultrasonography, CT, or MRI) and use of the electrode to generate thermal (radiofrequency) energy, which destroys the tumor. RFA can be performed percutaneously, laparoscopically, or during laparotomy.

While the use of RFA for liver metastases is reported to be effective and safe, there are currently no randomized data comparing resection and RFA. Abdalla et al. recently compared the results of operative resection versus RFA versus combined resection and RFA for colorectal liver metastases and found that recurrence was more common after RFA than after the combined procedure or resection alone (84%, 64%, and 52%, respectively). Moreover, true local recurrence (cut-edge of resected liver or RFA site) was more common after RFA than after resection (Fig. 10.4). Consequently, the long-term survival rate was higher after resection than after local ablation (65% vs. 22%). Given these findings, operative resection should be considered the treatment of choice for colorectal liver metastases, and use of RFA should be restricted mainly to patients in whom resection is not feasible technically.

Adjuvant Systemic and Regional Therapy

Recurrence after hepatic resection for colorectal liver metastases will occur in up to 70% of patients at some point during

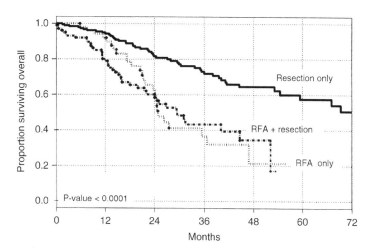

FIGURE 10.4. Overall survival of patients with colorectal liver metastases stratified by surgical treatment. Long-term survival was greatest in resected patients (Reprinted from Abdalla et al., 2004. With permission from Lippincott, Williams & Wilkins).

the course of their disease. Systemic chemotherapy is advocated to minimize these recurrences and prolong survival; however, the optimal strategy for systemic chemotherapy is yet to be defined.

The use of hepatic arterial infusion (HAI) as adjuvant treatment after hepatic resection has been investigated in several studies. HAI is attractive theoretically, because it allows infusion of a high dose of cytotoxic agents directly into the liver for both resectable and unresectable disease. HAI requires implantation of a catheter in the distal gastroduodenal artery and a pump in a subcutaneous pocket. Catheter and pump are usually placed during a laparotomy or, more recently, laparoscopically. Several studies have reported benefits with HAI; however, a recent systematic review from the Cochrane Collaboration looked at seven randomized trials of HAI of 592 patients and failed to find improvement in long-term survival with HAI. The review concluded that HAI reduces the rate of intrahepatic recurrence but does not prevent systemic extrahepatic metastases. HAI has not been investigated definitively in patients with unresectable colorectal liver metastases, and the available results are controversial.

Major efforts in basic research are focusing on identification of molecular pathways of malignant growth that can be disrupted by new biologic agents. Inhibitors of epidermal growth factor receptor and vascular endothelial growth factor receptor are under evaluation currently in international clinical trials, and their use appears to produce a survival advantage. Indeed, a recent randomized trial showed that addition of vascular endothelial growth factor receptor inhibitor (bevacizumab) to the fluorouracil-and irinotecan-based therapy resulted in clinically meaningful improvement in survival in patients with stage IV colon cancer. Such randomized controlled trials will be required to define the optimal use of chemotherapy after hepatic resection for colorectal liver metastases.

Resection of Non-Colorectal Liver Metastases

It is now widely accepted that liver resection is the only potentially curative therapy for colorectal liver metastases. In contrast, liver resection for non-colorectal metastases is performed infrequently, even though such resectional therapy can be performed safely and with low morbidity and mortality. Published reports on this approach report a heterogeneous series of patients, and, thus, drawing any conclusions on the basis of these reports is difficult.

Metastases from Neuroendocrine Neoplasms

Resection of functioning neuroendocrine liver metastases (NLM) reduces endocrine symptoms and prolongs survival. NLM have two main distinguishing features that provide the rationale for treating these metastases with hepatic resection: NLM usually grow slowly, and the survival of patients with NLM is longer than that of patients with other kinds of liver metastases. Moreover, endocrine activity can interfere seriously with patients' quality of life and also reduce long-term survival. Survival rates after resection of NLM are respectably high. Sarmiento et al. reported a 5-year survival rate of 61%, and Jaeck et al. reported a 3-year survival rate of 91%. In addition, operative resection results in control of symptoms of NLM in up to 90% of patients, even in cases of nonradical resection.

Alternative therapies for NLM include transarterial embolization (because NLM are hypervascular neoplasms) and administration of somatostatin analogs. Results of transarterial embolization have been encouraging, and somatostatin analogs may also reduce the release of neuroendocrine factors.

Metastases from Breast Cancer

Metastatic breast cancer is a systemic disease, and liver metastases from breast cancer are generally considered a poor prognostic factor, associated with a median survival of between 5 and 12 months. Although the indications for hepatic resection for breast metastases need to be further clarified, operative resection of breast liver metastases should be considered, but only as part of a multidisciplinary approach based mainly on systemic chemotherapy. In highly selected patients with liver metastases from breast cancer, complete resection of liver metastases (R0) in association with systemic cytotoxic, hormonal, and biologic therapies can produce 5-year overall and disease-free survival up to 61% and 31%, respectively. The most important prognostic factor appears to be a long disease-free interval between diagnosis of the primary breast cancer and diagnosis of liver metastases. In these patients, multiple hepatic metastases should be considered a relative contraindication for liver resection, while the presence of extrahepatic localization remains controversial.

Metastases from Other Types of Primary Neoplasms

There are a few single-institution studies reporting limited survival benefits after resection of liver metastases from melanoma, sarcoma, gynecologic, gastric, and pancreatic cancers. Indications for resection for these types of metastases are extremely limited, and no sufficient data are available to make any recommendation. The presence of liver metastases from gastrointestinal neoplasms other than colorectal cancer is a manifestation of diffuse disease and is usually associated with a grim prognosis.

Hepatic Transplantation for Metastatic Cancer of the Liver

Some groups have advocated a role for liver transplantation in the treatment of unresectable metastatic cancer of the liver, especially for the less aggressive metastatic neuroendocrine neoplasms. A limited number of patients have undergone liver transplantation for non-neuroendocrine liver metastases. Results have been generally disappointing – few patients have survived beyond 3 years.

Currently, most authors agree that given the limited number of patients who can be treated and the highrisk of recurrence because of the immunosuppressive therapy required after liver transplantation, liver transplantation has only a very limited role in the treatment of metastatic cancer of the liver. Moreover, the new, more aggressive, multimodality treatment strategies, such as neoadjuvant chemotherapy and two-stage hepatectomy with or without PVE, will allow us to offer hepatic resection with curative intent to more patients, meaning that fewer patients now have unresectable disease for which transplantation would even be considered.

Selected Readings

Abdalla EK, Vauthey JN, Ellis LM, et al. (2004) Recurrence and outcome following hepatic resection, radiofrequency ablation and combined resection/ablation for colorectal liver metastases. Ann Surg 239: 818–827

Abdalla EK, Denys A, Chevalier P, Nemr RA, Vauthey JN (2004) Total and segmental liver volume variations: implications for liver surgery. Surgery 135(4):404–410

Adam R, Delvart V, Pascal G, et al. (2004) Rescue surgery for unresectable colorectal liver metastases downstaged by chemotherapy. A model to predict long-term survival. Ann Surg 240:644–658

Aloia TA, Zorzi D, Abdalla EK, Vauthey JN (2005) Two-surgeon technique for hepatic parenchymal transaction using saline-linked cautery and ultrasonic dissection. Ann Surg 242(2):172–177

Bipat S, van Leeuwen MS, Coman EFI, et al. (2005) Colorectal liver metastases: CT, MR imaging, and PET for diagnosis - meta-analysis. Radiology 237:123–131

Domont J, Pawlik TM, Boige V, et al. (2005) Catalytic subunit of human telomerase reverse transcriptase is an independent predictor of survival in patients undergoing curative resection of hepatic colorectal metastasis: a mul-ticenter analysis. J Clin Oncol 23:3086–3093

Hurwitz H, Fehrenbacher L, Novotny W, et al. (2004) Bevacizumab plus irinotecan, fluorouracil, and leucovorin for metastatic colorectal cancer. N Engl J Med 350:2335–2342

Madoff DC, Abdalla EK, Vauthey JN (2005) Portal vein embolization in preparation for major hepatic resection: evolution of a new standard of care. J Vasc Interv Radiol 16:779–790

Pawlik TM, Scoggins CR, Zorzi D, et al. (2005) Effect of surgical margin status on survival and site of recurrence after hepatic resection for colorectal metastases. Ann Surg 241:715–724

Scheele J, Stangl R, Altendorf-Hofmann A (1990) Hepatic metastases from colorectal carcinoma: impact of surgical resection on the natural history. Br J Surg 77:1241–1246

Scheele J, Stang R, Altendorf-Hofmann A, et al. (1995) Resection of colorectal liver metastases. World J Surg 19:59–71

Vauthey JN, Pawlik TM, Ribero D, et al. (2006) Chemotherapy regimen predicts steatohepatitis and an increase in ninety-day mortality after surgery for hepatic colorectal metastases. J Clin Oncol 24:2065–2072

Part III
Biliary Benign

11
Postcholecystectomy Syndrome

Frank G. Moody

Pearls and Pitfalls

- Cholecystectomy is remarkably effective in relieving the symptoms associated with gallstones and other non-neoplastic diseases of the gallbladder.
- About 20% of patients who undergo cholecystectomy will experience symptoms similar to those for which they underwent operation.
- Recurrent episodes of upper abdominal pain is the most prominent feature of the postcholecystectomy syndrome.
- Patients at risk are those who have symptoms from diseases of the gastrointestinal tract (peptic ulcer disease, pancreatitis, reflux esophagitis, and irritable bowel syndrome) that were unrecognized preoperatively.
- There is a group of patients who have recurrent episodes of biliary or pancreatic-type pain after cholecystectomy, a retained stone within the common bile or cystic duct being one example.
- Pain from spasm of the sphincter of Oddi (biliary dyskinesia) may occur but is rare.
- Stenosing papillitis, while uncommon, can be a cause of unexplained postcholecystectomy pain.
- Medical drug addiction and drug seeking may be the problem.

K.I. Bland et al. (eds.), *Liver and Biliary Surgery*,
DOI 10.1007/978-1-84996-429-6_11,
© Springer-Verlag London Limited 2011

- All patients with postcholecystectomy pain should undergo a careful work-up before a therapeutic intervention.
- A transabdominal or endoscopic sphincterotomy with transampullary septectomy will be beneficial in about 70% of patients with stenosing papillitis, the problem is how to recognize who these patients are.
- It is likely that too many patients are having their papilla of Vater ablated or stented.
- Treat the papilla of Vater with great respect.

Background

While cholecystectomy is very effective in relieving the symptoms of diseases of the gallbladder, some patients (up to 20%) will continue to have or develop at a later date symptoms similar to those for which they had undergone cholecystectomy. Recurrent episodes of upper abdominal pain represent the clinical hallmark of this so-called postcholecystectomy syndrome. Gallstones are well tolerated in about half the patients who have them. It is the migration of the gallstones into the cystic duct (acute cholecystitis), bile duct (cholangitis), and through the papilla of Vater (biliary colic and acute pancreatitis) that reveals their presence and requires cholecystectomy for their resolution. In some patients (possibly many), gallstones are not the cause of the patients' problem. Some of the more common diseases that may mimic gallstones and therefore persist after cholecystectomy are listed in Table 11.1. The discussion below will focus on a small subset of patients who continue to have gallbladder-type pain after their gallbladder has been removed.

TABLE 11.1. Abdominal pain of nonbiliary origin.

Irritable bowel syndrome

Peptic ulcer disease

Reflux esophagitis

Pancreatitis

Coronary artery disease

Intercostal neuritis

TABLE 11.2. Postcholecystectomy pain of biliary origin.

Retained stone

Retained gallbladder

Cystic duct remnant with stone

Bile duct stricture

Stenosing papillitis

Several legitimate causes of the postcholecystectomy syndrome are listed in Table 11.2. Note that the list is short and that most of the problems on the list can be identified by readily available imaging techniques. A retained gallbladder, a retained stone within the cystic duct remnant or common bile duct, and a late stricture with biliary stones are all easy to characterize. Stenosing papillitis is the exception, because it is difficult to identify with confidence; when present, it can be treated successfully by total ablation of the anterior and posterior components of the papilla of Vater by either a transabdominal or transendoscopic approach by a procedure called a sphincteroplasty with transampullary septectomy.

Clinical Presentation

The typical patient with stenosing papillitis is a middle-aged female with recurrent episodes of upper abdominal pain months or years after cholecystectomy for gallstones or cholesterolosis. The pain is usually quite severe and requires a visit to the emergency room for relief by a narcotic analgesic. Liver and/or pancreatic serum markers are usually normal, as are imaging studies, including endoscopic retrograde cholangiopancreatography. Therein lies the problem. Fortunately, the illness is self-limited, usually subsiding within 1 day or 2, only to recur without warning weeks to months later. Such patients present a difficult management problem for their primary care physician, and often by the time they are referred to a surgeon who has treated such patients, they are addicted to narcotic analgesics. While in Salt Lake City in the 1970s, I became

TABLE 11.3. Clinical Characteristics of 28 postcholecystectomy patients treated by transabdominal sphincteroplasty and transampullary septectomy in Utah (1972–1976).

Female/male	23/5
Age (years)[a]	40
Postcholecystectomy (years)[a]	5.4
Duration of pain (years)[a]	5.3
Abstinence from alcohol	23
Prior choledochotomy	7
Prior sphincteroplasty	6
Psychiatric illness	6

[a]Mean.

interested in defining the cause of postcholecystectomy pain and initiated a study of such patients, characteristics of whom are listed in Table 11.3. The study population was unique, because the majority had complete abstinence from alcohol because of local custom. The majority were several years postcholecystectomy and had had recurrent episodes of pain for several years.

Diagnosis

Making a preoperative diagnosis of stenosing papillitis was a difficult task prior to the introduction of transendoscopic manometry. The diagnosis was presumptive and was based on a hunch from the history reinforced by an extensive work-up to exclude other disease processes and by office visits over a period of months to get to know the patient and his or her family situation. Consultations with a gastroenterologist, a psychiatrist, and experts in pain management are required.

The initial work-up should include a complete blood analysis of liver and pancreatic function, upper and lower gastrointestinal endoscopy, upper abdominal ultrasonography, abdominal computed tomography, endoscopic retrograde cholangiopancreatography, and a magnetic resonance cholangiopancreatogram if available. Unfortunately, this "million dollar work-up" may be non-revealing but must be carried out in a systematic manner in order not to miss other rare causes of recurrent abdominal pain, and also to raise the probability of a successful intervention when ablation of the papilla is undertaken.

Endoscopic transpapillary manometry is the most sensitive way to diagnose stenosing papillitis. Unfortunately, this test is not readily available in most communities and requires an individual with a special interest in its performance to be applied effectively. The essence of the test is a recording of increased static pressures within both the bile and the pancreatic ducts within the papilla as an indicator of a narrowed, fixed lumen within both these orifices.

Every effort should be made to detoxify the patient from analgesic dependency, but this attempt often fails. The patient must refrain from alcohol and smoking during this period of assessment and during attempts at medical management. This period of evaluation usually takes about 6 months. The patient has to earn an operative intervention, because even under the best of circumstances, an operative intervention, either by an open or a transendoscopic technique, will be empiric and must be offered with no guarantee of success.

Treatment

The only successful treatment for stenosing papillitis is total ablation of the papilla of Vater and its inherent sphincter of Oddi. This operation can be accomplished by either an open technique or by the transendoscopic route. The latter procedure requires someone highly specialized in advanced endoscopic surgery and therefore is not readily available in most medical communities. The procedure, termed a sphincteroplasty with transampullary septectomy, consists of a long, anterior sphincteroplasty (at least 15 mm) and transampullary septectomy.

The intent is to enlarge the orifice of both the bile duct and major pancreatic duct (duct of Wirsung) as they enter the duodenum. I will discuss the technical details of how I performed the procedure by the open technique on 115 patients prior to the availability of a transendoscopic approach. There were no hospital deaths and minimal morbidity. Hyperamylasemia occurred in about 10% of patients and was associated with clinical evidence of pancreatitis in only one patient.

The preoperative evaluation and preparation was as described above. Perioperative antibiotics are required. The abdomen should be opened through the incision used previously for the cholecystectomy. An upper midline incision is used for those who had undergone a laparoscopic cholecystectomy. Careful exploration of the abdomen is an essential feature of the operation, with special attention being paid to the organs within the upper abdomen, especially the pancreas and the bile duct. After fully Kocherizing the duodenum, the cystic duct remnant is identified and a filiform catheter (3 Fr) is passed through its apex into the duodenum. This maneuver allows easy identification of the papilla of Vater, which can be exposed through a small (3 cm) longitudinal duodenotomy. The anterior duodenal surface of the papilla is opened for about 15 mm, and the bile duct mucosa is secured to the duodenal mucosa at about 3 mm intervals with 5-0 polyglycolic acid (absorbable) sutures. Special care should be taken to approximate the apex of the incision. This maneuver completes the sphincteroplasty. The transampullary septum must then be excised. A headlight and magnifying loops are essential. Septectomy must be done with a high level of precision, because the septum is heavily scarred in most patients and must be removed completely to allow free egress of pancreatic juice. Tissue from both the anterior wall of the papilla and the transampullary septum should be submitted for pathologic examination. The epithelium of the duct of Wirsung is then approximated to the bile duct mucosa with 7-0, non-absorbable, single-strand, synthetic sutures. The papilla at the end of the procedure should reveal two widely patent and separate ostia for the bile and pancreatic ducts, as shown in Fig. 11.1.

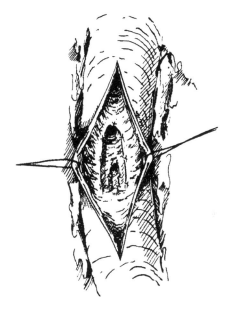

FIGURE 11.1. A schematic representation of the orifices of the bile duct and duct of Wirsung within the posterior wall of the duodenum after a sphincteroplasty and transampullary septectomy. Note that both the anterior as well as the posterior wall of the bile duct within the papilla of Vater have been excised, and that the bile duct to duodenal mucosa and pancreatic duct to bile duct mucosa has been approximated precisely with fine, interrupted sutures as described in the text (From Moody et al., 1983. With permission of Lippincott, Williams & Wilkins).

Outcome

I performed the operation as described above on 115 patients over a 20-year period. The first 28 patients represented a homogeneous cohort of non-alcoholic postcholecystectomy patients who were studied carefully over a 5-to 15-year period. Many patients were chemically dependent on narcotic analgesics. Surprisingly, 75% were rendered pain free over this time period. The remainder of the patients represented a more varied population, which included social drinkers and

TABLE 11.4. Outcome after sphincteroplasty and transampullary septectomy in 83 patients with postcholecystectomy syndrome followed
for 1–10 years.

Status of papilla	Results		
	Good	Fair	Poor
Papillitis	15	16	9
Septitis[a]	17	10	9
Normal	4	1	2
Total	36 (43%)	27 (33%)	20 (24%)

[a]*Disease limited to septum.*

a variety of reoperative cases following my move to Houston,
Texas. Much to my surprise, at a 1-to 10-year follow-up, the
results were equivalent to those obtained in the more selective population of the index group from Utah (Table 11.4).
The best results were obtained in patients who had well-
documented gallstone disease prior to operation. The worse
results were obtained in patients in whom the procedure on
the papilla was performed simultaneously with a cholecystectomy. Poor results were also obtained in patients with cholesterolosis of the papilla possibly as a consequence of the
extensive inflammation in and around the papilla in this
entity. The best results occurred in patients who had a
transampullary septectomy after failing to gain pain relief
from an adequate anterior sphincteroplasty. Ten of 115
patients had pancreas divisum in addition to extensive stenosis
of the papilla of Vater. Possibly, they also benefited from the
pupilloplasty, because their results were comparable to the
overall group, but the benefit may have related to the simultaneous surgical enlargement of the duct of Santorini in this
population. What is not clear is why about 10% of patients
that had no demonstrable pathology of the papilla also had a
result comparable to the overall group (71% pain relief).
Possibly their abdominal pain was a consequence of spasm of
the sphincter of Oddi (biliary dyskinesia).

It is likely that we as surgeons will not be asked to treat
non-neoplastic diseases of the papilla in the future, because

gastroenterologists have adopted this organ as one of special interest to them. There is some concern that papillary disease is being over diagnosed and treated. I am convinced that stenosing papillitis does exist, that it is a consequence of injury from chronic passage of gallstones, and on rare occasions, that it is the site of inflammation from cholesterolosis. Earlier operative intervention by minimal invasive means (laparoscopic cholecystectomy) in symptomatic gallstone disease should have a beneficial effect on the incidence of papillary disease with less injury from the chronic passage of gallstones. If this is true, then postcholecystectomy pain from stenosing papillitis in the future will be only of historic interest. In the interim, we should treat the papilla of Vater with great respect and only approach it surgically as a last resort in the management of postcholecystectomy pain.

Selected Readings

Baille J (2005) Sphincter of Oddi dysfunction; overdue for an overhaul. Am J Gastroenterol 100:1217

Moody FG, Becker JM, Potts JR (1983) Transduodenal sphincteroplasty and transampullary septectomy for postcholecystectomy pain. Ann Surg 197:627–636

Moody FG (1985) Pathogenesis and treatment of inflamma-tory lesions of the papilla of Vater. Jpn J Surg 15:341–347

Moody FG, Calabuig R, Vecchio R, Runkel N (1990) Stenosis of the sphincter of Oddi. Surg Clin North Am 70:1341–1354

Moody FG, Kwong K (2002) Postcholecystectomy syn-drome, Chapter 102. In: Bland KI (ed) The practice of general surgery. W.B. Saunders, Philadelphia, pp 653–658

Piccini G (2004) Diagnosing and treating sphincter of Oddi dysfunction: a critical literature review and re-evaluation. J Clin Gastroenterol 38:350–359

Ponsky TA, DeSagun R, Brody F, et al. (2005) Surgical therapy for biliary dyskinesia: a meta-analysis and review of the literature. J Laparoendosc Adv Surg Tech A 15:439

Touli J, Di Francesco V, Saccone G, et al. (1996) Division of the sphincter of Oddi for treatment of dysfunction associated with recurrent pancreatitis. Br J Surg 83:1205–1210

12
Asymptomatic Gallstones

Robert V. Rege

Pearls and Pitfalls

- Asymptomatic ("silent") gallstones are much more common than appreciated 40 years ago, due to improvements in imaging.
- The great majority of patients with asymptomatic gallstones remain so for extended periods of time.
- Patients with symptomatic gallstones are likely to have recurrent symptoms and to develop complications of gallstone disease.
- Patients with mildly symptomatic gallstones act more like asymptomatic, as compared to symptomatic patients.
- Most patients with asymptomatic gallstones are best treated expectantly (observed until they develop symptoms).
- Select groups of patients, including patients with gallstones and hemolytic anemia, children, and patients with large (>2.5 cm) stones, may benefit from prophylactic or incidental cholecystectomy.
- Incidental cholecystectomy at the time of another abdominal operation may be of benefit, because patients are more likely to develop symptomatic disease and complications after their primary operation, and cholecystectomy does not appear to increase the morbidity and mortality for most operations.

K.I. Bland et al. (eds.), *Liver and Biliary Surgery*,
DOI 10.1007/978-1-84996-429-6_12,
© Springer-Verlag London Limited 2011

- Prophylactic cholecystectomy is not recommended currently for diabetic patients, cirrhotic patients, or patients undergoing solid organ transplantation.

In the United States alone, about 600,000 patients undergo cholecystectomy annually for symptoms or complications caused by gallstones, although more than a million patients develop gallstones each year. Therefore, many more patients harbor gallstones than require treatment, and consequently, large numbers of individuals exist in the population with asymptomatic (or "silent") gallstone disease. Recent data indicate that the indications for cholecystectomy have liberalized since the introduction of laparoscopic cholecystectomy. For example, the relative proportion of cholecystectomies in relation to other operations increased from about 13% of all operations throughout 1990–1994 to 22% during 1995–2001. The reasons for these changes are unknown but may represent the willingness of physicians to recommend operation, and patients to accept recommendation, with less or no symptoms. During the same period of time, there has been no changes in the morbidity or mortality of the operation.

This chapter outlines our current understanding of the natural history of asymptomatic gallstones and the frequency of developing symptoms or complications if patients with silent gallstones are observed and treated nonoperatively. Recommendations for treatment of patients with asymptomatic gallstones, including special subgroups of patients, are based on our current understanding of the risk/ benefit ratio of operation versus non-operation.

Historical Perspective

Gallstone disease is one of the most common disorders affecting mankind. In Western countries, cholesterol gallstones predominate, while in the remainder of the world pigment stones are more common. Although types of gallstones differ, the incidence of gallstones is similar worldwide. Gallstone prevalence varies with gender (11–15% of women and 3–11% of men), increasing age, and multiple pregnancies. There is also a

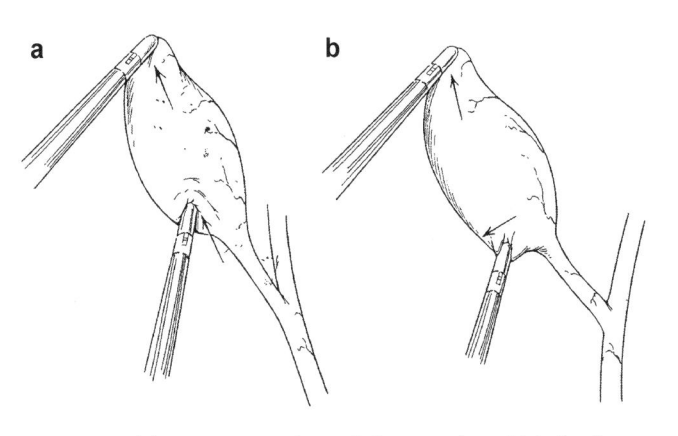

FIGURE 13.1. (**a**) Demonstration of the way in which inadvertent traction caudally of the gallbladder and infundibulum narrows the angle between the cystic and hepatic ducts thereby making it more likely that these ducts will be misidentified. (**b**) Appropriate displacement of Hartmann's Pouch laterally opens the angle between the cystic and hepatic ducts.

reduce the risk of BDI. He has stressed the importance of identifying the cystic duct at its junction with the gallbladder and of avoiding inappropriate traction of the gallbladder superiorly since this may give the surgeon the false impression that the common bile duct represents the cystic duct (Fig. 13.1). His described principles have been adopted by the Society of American Gastrointestinal and Endoscopic Surgeons (Table 13.1). Strasberg has also highlighted the importance of the conclusive identification of the cystic duct and artery. The "critical view of safety" (Fig. 13.2) which he describes, requires that only two structures are connected to the lowest part of the gallbladder when its attachment to the liver bed has been freed. Despite such recommendations, we have observed in referred patients, BDI associated with major portal vein injury thought to be due to bleeding from the middle hepatic vein above and BDI associated with injury to the pancreas and pancreatic duct inferiorly. Similarly, we have managed patients whose cholecystectomy passed without apparent difficulty and yet presented postoperatively with complications resulting proportion of such cases resulting in litigious action against the surgeon. Despite these known facts, there remain significant delays in specialist referral and, in the United Kingdom, patients continue to undergo attempted repair by inexperienced surgeons.

Cause of Bile Duct Injury

It is accepted widely that major bile duct injury results as a direct consequence of misinterpretation of the biliary anatomy by the surgeon during surgery. Following the introduction of laparoscopic cholecystectomy, bile duct injury tended to occur early in the experience of the surgeon and was attributed to the "learning curve". However, since then the technique has become very well established and it is now clear that the experience of the surgeon does not safeguard against bile duct injury. One third of BDI are committed by surgeons who have performed over 200 laparoscopic cholecystectomies and one third of all surgeons in the United States have injured the bile duct during LC on at least one occasion. Although bile duct injury is not an uncommon experience, this complication should be regarded as entirely avoidable.

Prevention of Bile Duct Injury

Attempts to determine those specific pitfalls that might occur during laparoscopic cholecystectomy resulting in BDI have demonstrated technical failure and lack of knowledge contribute to only a small proportion of cases. The principle cause is misinterpretation of the biliary anatomy when the CBD is mistaken for the cystic duct. Reviewed operation notes during which BDI has occurred often describe the procedure as "straightforward". As a consequence, two thirds of BDI are not recognized at the time of surgery leading to a delay in diagnosis which is associated with a less favorable prognosis for consequent repair. Importantly, Hunter has made a number of technical recommendations, which if adhered to closely, may

Choledocholithiasis: Up to 10% of patients with cholelithiasis present with simultaneous choledocholithiasis, with an increasing incidence in the elderly. In most cases, the choledocholithiasis is of gallbladder origin, having migrated through the cystic duct. Primary choledocholithiasis, defined as common bile duct stones occurring >2 years after cholecystectomy, can also occur, being formed during periods of stasis within the CBD.

Patients with associated choledocholithiasis present typically with intense upper quadrant pain, usually more epigastric, acute jaundice, and dark urine (bilirubinuria). Hepatic function tests may demonstrate increased serum concentrations of total and conjugated bilirubin, alkaline phosphatase activity, and aspartate transaminase activities. Findings on US may include visualization of the choledocholithiasis (and usually cholelithiasis) or related signs, such as CBD dilation >7 mm or a dilated cystic duct. Given the low sensitivity of US for choledocholithiasis, in patients where a high suspicion exists, MRCP provides a non-invasive, highly sensitive adjunct to make the diagnosis. In patients in whom choledocholithiasis is suspected strongly on US, MRCP is probably not worthwhile, because MRCP cannot treat choledocholithiasis; in this clinical situation, ERCP with endoscopic interventional techniques of choledocholithiasis retrieval seems most efficient and cost-effective.

Open cholecystectomy with choledochotomy and T-tube choledochostomy was, for many years, the operative approach for choledocholithiasis. At present, the favored approach is the use of ERCP with endoscopic sphincterotomy/stone extraction for management of the choledocholithiasis prior to or after laparoscopic cholecystectomy. In some centers, laparoscopic cholecystectomy and laparoscopic CBD exploration and stone removal has been reported with success but requires considerable experience.

Cholelithiasis and gallbladder cancer: As stated above, virtually all patients with gallbladder cancer have cholelithiasis. Associated gallbladder cancer should be suspected with polyps >1.5 cm, non-mobile "stones," eccentric thickening of the wall of the gallbladder, or extrahepatic biliary obstruction beginning at the entrance of the cystic duct. In patients with cholelithiasis and radiographic suspicion of gallbladder cancer, initial laparoscopic exploration is useful for identifying lymph node infiltration and metastasis, followed by open cholecystectomy with oncologic resection of adjacent liver and regional lymph nodes if indicated.

Cholelithiasis and cirrhosis of the liver: Prevalence of gallstones (pigment stones) is increased among patients with cirrhosis. Operative intervention in these patients, however, is associated with increased risk of perioperative complications, especially in the presence of portal hypertension. As a combined morbidity and mortality of 30% occurs after open cholecystectomy, any intervention should be considered carefully, especially in patients with Child's A or B cirrhosis or those with portal hypertension. Laparoscopic cholecystectomy should still be the treatment of choice among patients with cirrhosis; however, the rate of conversion to an open procedure is higher among these patients.

Cholelithiasis and pregnancy: Symptomatic cholelithiasis is not uncommon during pregnancy or in the early postpartum period. Lu et al. reviewed 78 pregnant patients with symptomatic cholelithiasis and found that 55% of patients had uncomplicated disease, 26% developed acute cholecystitis, 15% had associated gallstone pancreatitis, and 4% had associated choledocholithiasis. Elective cholecystectomy in pregnant patients with cholelithiasis is still controversial, although evidence suggests that it is relatively safe in the second and early third trimester and decreases gallstone-related complications which may occur prior to delivery. When indicated during pregnancy, cholecystectomy is recommended during the second trimester, where the risk to mother and fetus are less, avoiding first semester miscarriage or concerns of mutagenic effects of the anesthetic and third semester premature birth.

Porcelain gallbladder: Calcification of the gallbladder wall secondary to the chronic inflammation of cholelithiasis is known as *porcelain gallbladder*. It is an uncommon entity and presents in fewer than 1% of patients with cholelithiasis. Porcelain gallbladder is typically asymptomatic. Studies held in the 1960s suggested a correlation between porcelain gallbladder and gallbladder cancer of 12–61%. Recent studies, however, have challenged the validity of this correlation; nevertheless, cholecystectomy is typically recommended. The term "porcelain gallbladder" has several meanings. Heavy, thick, platelike calcification is not associated with gallbladder cancer, but punctate mucosal calcifications are a definite risk marker of gallbladder carcinoma and should be an indication for cholecystectomy, even in the asymptomatic patient.

Selected Readings

Berger M, Van der Velden J, Lijmer J, et al. (2000) Abdominal symptoms: do they predict gallstones? A systematic review. Scand J Gastroenterol 35:70–76

Ji W, Li L, Wang Z, et al. (2005) A randomized controlled trial of laparoscopic versus open cholecystectomy in patients with cirrhotic portal hypertension. World J Gas-troenterol 11:2513–2517

Lu E, Curet M, El-Sayed Y, Kirkwood K, (2004) Medical versus surgical management of biliary tract disease in pregnancy. Am J Surg 188:755–759

Miquel JF, Covarrubias C, Villarroel L, et al. (1998) Genetic epidemiology of cholesterol cholelithiasis among Chilean Hispanic, Amerindians and Maoris. Gastroenterology 115:937–946

Nakeeb A, Comuzzie A, Martin L, et al. (2002) Gallstones: genetics versus environment. Ann Surg 235:842–849

Nathanson LK, O'Rourke NA, Martin IJ, et al. (2005) Post-operative ERCP versus laparoscopic choledocotomy for clearance of selected bile duct calculi: a randomized trial. Ann Surg 242:188–192

Stephen AE, Berger DL, (2001) Carcinoma in the porcelain gallbladder: a relationship revisited. Surgery 129:699–703

Yeh C, Chen M, Jan Y, (2002) Laparoscopic cholecystectomy in 226 cirrhotic patients. Experience of a single center in Taiwan. Surg Endosc 16:1583–1587

15
Choledocholithiasis

**Toshiyuki Mori, Yutaka Suzuki, Masanori Sugiyama,
and Yutaka Atomi**

Pearls and Pitfalls

- Choledocholithiasis may be identified in 5–10% of patients undergoing elective cholecystectomy.
- The presence of choledocholithiasis correlates with patient age and is: 5%, 15%, and 35% in patients <60, 60–79, and >80 years of age, respectively.
- Common duct stones can be classified into two types: primary and secondary. Primary stones form *de novo* in the common duct as a result of biliary infection or stasis. Secondary stones are identical in composition to gallbladder stones and presumably migrate from the gallbladder.
- Clinical features of bile duct stones range from an incidental finding discovered during cholecystectomy to acute suppurative cholangitis.
- An increased serum alkaline phosphatase activity, jaundice, and a dilated common bile duct are characteristic signs of common duct stones, but are not specific.
- Magnetic resonance cholangiopancreatography (MRCP) is an effective, noninvasive method for detecting choledocholithiasis when suspected.
- Endoscopic retrograde cholangiopancreatography (ERCP) with sphincterotomy and stone retrieval is a safe and effective treatment of common duct stones.

K.I. Bland et al. (eds.), *Liver and Biliary Surgery*,
DOI 10.1007/978-1-84996-429-6_15,
© Springer-Verlag London Limited 2011

- When technically possible, laparoscopic, transcystic common bile duct exploration with stone retrieval is a safe and effective treatment option in experienced centers.

Overall, 5–15% of patients undergoing cholecystectomy for cholelithiasis have concomitant bile duct stones, and a small percentage of patients after cholecystectomy will develop common duct stones. Thus, bile duct stones and their management constitute an important clinical problem. Traditionally, laparotomy with common duct exploration was the primary therapy since the performance of the first successful biliary lithotomy by Courvoisier in 1890. The introduction of endoscopic sphincterotomy by Classen and Kawai in 1974 initiated a change in the management of retained and recurrent bile duct stones. Advances in endoscopic equipment, techniques, and the availability of skilled endoscopists have solidified the success of this minimally invasive treatment option. Today, open common duct exploration is rarely necessary in most centers. Laparoscopic common duct exploration has also been described and is gaining popularity in several centers. Furthermore, modern imaging modalities, including MRI, multidetector CT, and endoscopic ultrasonography (EUS), have allowed improved detection of choledocholithiasis. At present, it would be difficult to set a universally accepted algorithm for the diagnosis and treatment of common bile duct stone due to a wide variety of highly accurate imaging modalities and varying expertise of biliary endoscopists and laparoscopic surgeons. Although prospective studies comparing these newer methods to older standards of diagnosis are not reported in the literature, this chapter will discuss the current diagnosis and treatment of choledocholithiasis.

Definition, Classification, and Pathogenesis

Common duct stones are defined as calculi in the common duct regardless of the coexistence of stones in the gallbladder. When stones are present proximal to the confluence of the right and left hepatic ducts, they are termed intrahepatic. Bile duct stones can be classified into two types, depending on their site of origin: primary stones form de novo in the bile duct (after cholecystectomy), whereas secondary stones are presumed to have migrated from the gallbladder into the biliary tree.

Primary common duct stones are composed predominantly of calcium bilirubinate monomers with variable, but minor quantities of cholesterol, and calcium soaps of fatty acids such as calcium palmitate. These stones are often described as "earthy," brownish yellow, and are usually very soft and friable. Their pathogenesis is attributed to two main factors: bacterial infection and biliary stasis. The predominant organisms isolated from bile in the presence of primary bile duct stones include gram-negative enteric organisms such as *Escherichia coli* and *Klebsiella* species, and anaerobes, such as *Bacteroides* and *Clostridium*. These bacteria secrete enzymes such as β-glucuronidase that catalyze the conjugation of bilirubin and the lysis of phospholipids, leading to deposition of calcium bilirubinate and calcium palmitate. Bacterial digestion of bile salts and lecithin further promotes lithogenesis and adds cholesterol to the primary duct stones. The association of biliary strictures and severe ductal dilation with the formation of brown pigment stones supports the contributory role of biliary stasis in the pathogenesis of primary duct stones. Finally, foreign objects, such as nonabsorbable suture material and hemostatic clips, have also been associated with primary duct stone formation, presumably by providing a nidus for bacterial colonization and subsequent stone growth.

Secondary stones are identical in composition to stones in the gallbladder (predominantly cholesterol in 80% or black pigment in 20%) and are presumed to form in the gallbladder with subsequent migration into the biliary tree. The events predisposing to this migration remain unknown; however, the diameter of the cystic duct appears to be important. In a prospective evaluation of 331 patients undergoing cholecystectomy, stones present in the gallbladder could be advanced manually through the cystic duct in 60% of patients with concomitant common bile duct stones, in 67% with gallstone pancreatitis, but in only 3% of those with gallstones alone.

None of the gallstones with diameters greater than the diameter of the cystic duct could be forced through it. Rarely, large gallstones (unable to traverse the cystic duct) can enter the bile duct through a fistula.

Prevalence

The prevalence of common duct stones is reportedly 5–15% of patients undergoing cholecystectomy for cholelithiasis. Several series have demonstrated a correlation between age and the presence of common duct stones. For patients aged <60, 60–79, and >75 years undergoing cholecystectomy for cholecystolithiasis, concomitant choledocholithiasis has been identified in 5%, 15%, and 35%, respectively. One theory for this relationship with age is the time at risk for choledocholithiasis in patients with cholelithiasis.

Stones discovered in the bile ducts after cholecystectomy are defined as retained, residual, or recurrent. When choledocholithiasis is identified by cholangiography shortly after cholecystectomy, they are termed "retained," because these stones are missed during the operation. Stones that are found later (<2 years after cholecystectomy) and contain the same composition (black pigment or cholesterol) as the gallbladder stones are termed "residual" stones. Stones that form within the bile duct (primary duct stones, brown stones) or those discovered >2 years after the cholecystectomy are termed "recurrent" stones and are assumed to be primary common duct stones. Analysis of composition of 56 sets of common duct stones revealed that most stones (75%) found at, or shortly after, cholecystectomy were of the cholesterol or black pigment type. In contrast, the majority discovered 21 months or more after cholecystectomy were brown pigment stones. The prevalence of either retained stones or residual stones is estimated to be 1–7% and 2–5%, respectively. With the assumption that some patients with choledocholithiasis may remain asymptomatic, the actual prevalence of retained common bile duct stones may be greater.

Clinical Features

The spectrum of clinical features of choledocholithiasis ranges from an incidental finding during cholecystectomy to acute suppurative cholangitis. Whereas the overall prevalence of common duct stones discovered at the time of cholecystectomy is about 10%, the proportion that is unsuspected (normal laboratory data and normal bile duct by ultrasonography) is probably 1–3%. The patient with choledocholithiasis commonly has severe discomfort in the epigastrium or right upper quadrant that often radiates to the back and may be associated with nausea and vomiting. The pain presents as discrete attacks lasting 30 min to several hours and is indistinguishable from pain elicited by gallstone impaction in the cystic duct, except for its often epigastric location. These symptoms may occur at any time and are not necessarily related to food ingestion. Ductal stones can cause obstruction to bile flow, pain, obstructive jaundice, and infection/cholangitis. The classic triad of right upper quadrant pain, fever and chills, and jaundice, termed "Charcot's triad," is present in 50–75% of patients with acute cholangitis. When patients exhibit hypotension and mental confusion in addition to Charcot's triad, it is termed Reynald's pentad and portends a high mortality of 30–50%.

Gallstone pancreatitis is a potential serious sequela of choledocholithiasis. While most common bile duct stones that cause pancreatitis pass spontaneously, the severity of the illness is related generally to the severity of the pancreatitis, ranging from mild and self-limited to severe and necrotizing, with the complications of infection, peripancreatic fluid collections, and death. Acute cholangitis may accompany the pancreatitis and worsens the prognosis.

Laboratory Examination

Several serum laboratory tests are helpful in the evaluation of patients with suspected choledocholithiasis. These tests reflect the degree of biliary tract obstruction; however, they may be normal in patients with non-obstructing stones. The alkaline phosphatase activity is probably the most sensitive measure of obstruction and is usually increased twofold to fivefold in choledocholithiasis. Higher levels may be suggestive of a more chronic, malignant biliary obstruction. Increased serum bilirubin concentration adds specificity to the laboratory diagnosis of bile duct obstruction and is present in 50–75% of symptomatic patients with choledocholithiasis. Of the patients with acute cholecystitis but without choledocholithiasis, 30% will have hyperbilirubinemia (usually <3 mg/dl). A serum bilirubin concentration of >7 mg/dl in patients with acute cholecystitis usually indicates concomitant bile duct stones. Marked increase in serum bilirubin (>10 mg/dl) in the absence of suppurative cholangitis suggests malignant obstruction or concomitant parenchymal disease of the liver. Only rarely does choledocholithiasis cause a complete and progressive biliary obstruction. Fluctuation of the serum bilirubin level may also suggest choledocholithiasis.

The ability of aspartate aminotransferase activity to differentiate biliary obstruction due to calculi from that due to malignant neoplasm has been suggested. With choledocholithiasis, the serum level often increases acutely to 3–5 times normal and may increase into the thousands (hepatitis range), but typically returns rapidly toward normal. This phenomenon is not seen with malignant obstruction.

When superimposed biliary infection occurs, the white cell count is increased usually to 15,000–18,000 mm^{-3} but can also be decreased markedly to 2,000–3,000 mm^{-3} with overwhelming sepsis. Patients who are asymptomatic or who present with biliary colic frequently have a normal white cell count.

Imaging Studies

Ultrasonography (Fig. 15.1). The sensitivity of transcutaneous ultrasonography in detecting choledocholithiasis is low, but is fairly specific. In patients with a dilated common bile duct, choledocholithiasis or other causes of obstruction are inferred; however, 30% of patients with choledocholithiasis have no

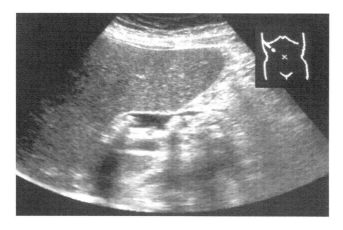

FIGURE 15.1. Although ultrasonography may only delineate dilation of the common bile duct, stones are imaged in only about 15% of patients with choledocholithiasis.

evidence of ductal dilation on ultrasonography. Although able to assess accurately biliary dilation, ultrasonography is able to detect common bile duct stones in only 15% of patients. This sensitivity increases to 33% in patients who are jaundiced, but this overall low sensitivity requires other imaging modalities in the majority of patients with suspected choledocholithiasis.

Intravenous cholangiography. Intravenous cholangiography was used historically in the detection of choledocholithiasis, but fell into disfavor because of its low sensitivity and potential for adverse reactions. In a recent study, however, preoperative intravenous cholangiograms were obtained in 100 consecutive patients undergoing laparoscopic cholecystectomy; all patients had subsequent operative cholangiography. Intravenous cholangiography identified choledocholithiasis in eight patients with only one false-positive result. Operative cholangiography discovered only one additional patient with choledocholithiasis. Only two patients had mild reactions to the contrast agent. If the results of this study are verified, intravenous cholangiography may be of value in the detection of common duct stones before laparoscopic surgery.

MRCP (Fig. 15.2). MR imaging has seen a rapid technologic development in recent years, with dramatic improvement in noninvasive techniques and diagnostic accuracy for both abdominal imaging and MRCP. For MRCP, the combination of T_1-and T_2-weighted thin section scans in coronal oblique planes together with thick slab radial cholangiographic T_2-weighted images to delineate anatomy are obtained. MR has proven to be an excellent, noninvasive, accurate imaging technique without the need for ionizing radiation or, in many cases, the need for any type of oral or intravenously infused contrast administration. Moreover, MR imaging is relatively operator-independent and has no or negligible morbidity. The most commonly used contrast agent is a gadolinium chelate, which has excellent patient safety and tolerability. In one study, MRCP was performed in 202 patients with a suspicion of choledocholithiasis based on clinical presentation and/or cholestatic liver function tests. ERCP was performed subsequently in all patients in whom MRCP indicated choledocholithiasis, as well as in those patients with a strong clinical suspicion of choledocholithiasis despite a negative MRCP. In 25 patients, MRCP suggested choledocholithiasis, which was proven subsequently with ERCP in 24 patients. Despite a negative MRCP, 27 additional patients had a subsequent ERCP, none of whom had evidence of stones. In the entire group, MRCP resulted in a 100% sensitivity and a 96% specificity in detecting stones in the common bile duct. In obstructive jaundice, MRCP has an overall accuracy of 96–100% for demonstrating the anatomic level of obstruction and a 90% accuracy for the cause of obstruction. MRCP may, therefore, be able to replace diagnostic ERCP in patients with suspected choledocholithiasis, while the more invasive ERCP may be reserved for patients requiring endoscopic intervention.

The limitations of MR imaging are due predominantly to the difficulty in imaging certain groups of patients, such as those with claustrophobia or those with cardiac pacemakers. MR imaging is also not suitable when therapeutic intervention is planned.

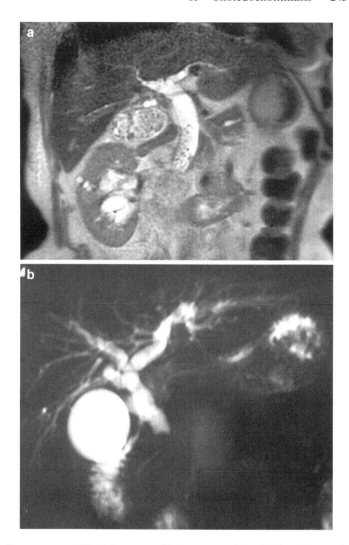

FIGURE 15.2. MRCP has a sensitivity approaching 99% and a specificity of 96% in detecting CBD stones and has become the method
of choice when available. (**a**) Multiple small common bile duct stones.
(**b**) Obstructive jaundice due to CBD stone.

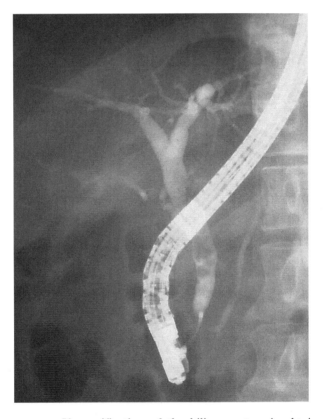

FIGURE 15.3. If opacification of the biliary system is obtained, endoscopic retrograde cholangiography (ERC) has a sensitivity approaching 100% in the detection of obstruction. As MRCP has become more widely available for detecting common duct stones, ERC is reserved for endoscopic intervention.

ERC and percutaneous transhepatic cholangiograms (Fig. 15.3). Percutaneous transhepatic cholangiography (PTC) provides direct imaging of the biliary tree and remains the gold standard in depicting subtle changes within the bile ducts and in the detection of small calculi. If opacification of the biliary system is obtained, cholangiography has a sensitivity approaching 100% in the detection of obstruction. ERCP is now performed more often than PTC. Both approaches of direct ductal imaging are invasive investigations which are operator-dependent and have a relatively high morbidity of 1–7% for ERCP and 3–5% for PTC. ERCP has a sensitivity of 90–96% and specificity of 98% in detecting choledocholithiasis, but in 3–10% of patients, cannulation of the bile duct is unsuccessful. PTC provides excellent imaging with a success rate of up to 99%, although this level of success is highly dependent on the presence of biliary dilation. As the diagnostic role of MRCP evolves, the main advantages of ERCP and PTC are primarily in their therapeutic use with the ability to extract stones, perform tissue biopsy, and replace stents.

Endoscopic ultrasonography. EUS offers a diagnostic accuracy comparable to that of MRCP; however, the invasive nature, operator dependence, and restricted availability have limited its widespread use in detection of choledocholithiasis.

Management

The primary goal in the management of choledocholithiasis is to obtain complete clearance of the common duct and cholecystectomy, when indicated. In patients with suppurative cholangitis or gallstone pancreatitis, control of infection and inflammation is a prerequisite. When first introduced, endoscopic sphincterotomy was utilized primarily in elderly, high-risk patients with recurrent choledocholithiasis. With the greater availability of biliary endoscopists, technical improvements in instrumentation, and more extensive experience, the performance of sphincterotomy in the treatment of choledocholithiasis has broadened considerably.

Endoscopic Intervention

With technologic advancements, endoscopic intervention as a primary treatment of choledocholithiasis is performed with increasing frequency. Although randomized, controlled trials comparing endoscopic intervention with other treatments are lacking, endoscopic sphincterotomy has become the procedure of choice in virtually all patients with recurrent choledocholithiasis. The technique uses a side-viewing endoscope, a catheter with 20–30 mm of wire exposed at the distal end (sphincterotome), and electrodiathermy to incise the papilla and the sphincter muscle fibers that surround the ampulla of Vater and distal common bile duct (sphincter choledochus). The incision is made in the 11 o'clock to 12 o'clock direction along the longitudinal fold by lifting the wire in this direction while applying current through the wire (Fig. 15.4a). A 10–15 mm sphincterotomy is made, although the length of the sphincter-otomy should be tailored to the size of the stones, the length of the longitudinal fold, and the diameter of the distal common bile duct. The average bile duct stone is 8–10 mm, so most stones can be extracted with a balloon or basket

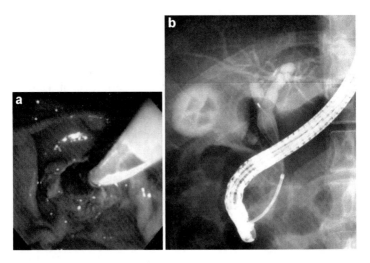

FIGURE 15.4. Endoscopic intervention. (a) Endoscopic sphincterotomy. The incision is made in the 11 o'clock to 12 o'clock direction along the longitudinal fold by lifting the wire in this direction while applying current through the wire. A 10–15 mm incision is then made. (b) Stone removal. A basket or balloon catheter is introduced for stone retrieval.

after routine sphincterotomy (Fig. 15.4b). The success rate for sphincterotomy is 90–95%, and the success rate for stone extraction is 90–95%. When performed by experienced biliary endoscopists, the overall success for complete ductal clearance is in the range of 85–90%.

Endoscopic sphincterotomy has a complication rate of about 8% and a mortality rate of about 1%; however, in elderly, high-risk patients, major complication rates are as high as 19% with mortality rates of up to 8%. Major complications include bleeding, perforation, infection, pancreatitis, and basket impaction, and operative intervention may be required in 20% of these patients. Given these potential risks and the unknown long-term effects of sphincterotomy, several authors have suggested that sphincterotomy should be avoided in patients with "small stones" that can be removed with papillary balloon dilatation or administration of smooth muscle relaxants (nitroglycerin).

Failure to achieve bile duct clearance may occur for a variety of reasons. Inability to advance the endoscope to the papilla may occur as a result of esophageal or duodenal stricture. Reaching the papilla endoscopically is difficult or impossible in patients with a Roux-en-Y gastrojejunostomy. For difficult anatomic situations in which the papilla is not obvious, a transhepatically placed wire may be passed antegrade down the common bile duct, and into the duodenum, and grasped by the endoscopic forceps, allowing the endoscope to be pulled up to the papilla (the so-called rendezvous technique). Cannulation of the papilla may be difficult in the setting of papillary stenosis or periampullary diverticulum. In patients with Billroth II anatomy, successful cannulation has been achieved in 46–89% of patients and may be influenced by the type of anastomosis. ERCP was performed successfully in one series in 64% of patients with a retrocolic gastroenterostomy and a short afferent limb, but could be done in only 33% of patients with an antecolic gastroenterostomy with a longer afferent limb.

Intraoperative cholangiography during laparoscopic cholecystectomy may reveal unexpected common bile duct stones.

In such cases, a 16-gauge catheter can be introduced in the common bile duct via the cystic duct. This catheter can be used postoperatively as a route for direct cholangiography. When common duct stones are found, endoscopic sphinctero-tomy and stone extraction is indicated. In cases where cannula-tion of the papilla is unsuccessful, a guide wire can be passed through the catheter into the duodenum and the sphincter choledochus can be intubated and cut. Deep cannulation over or along this guide wire can be done easily.

Large stones are difficult to capture by a basket, and therefore, fragmentation of the stone by intracorporeal or extracorporeal lithotripsy may be necessary. Fragmentation can be achieved in such cases by delivering a shockwave directly onto the surface of stone with either a flexible elec-trohydraulic probe or by using a flexible quartz fiber to deliver light from a laser. More recently, mechanical litho-triptor-wire baskets capable of trapping stones and exerting sufficient force to break (or disrupt) most bile duct stones have become available. Mechanical lithotripsy yields frag-mentation rates between 27% and 100%, including "giant" stones with diameters >2 cm.

Long-Term Endobiliary Stenting

Long-term endobiliary stenting is a potential palliative option in elderly, high-risk patients with non-extractable bile duct stones. A stent is placed so that one limb is above the stone and the other limb is inside the duodenum. Although stents often occlude within months, long-term biliary drainage is maintained, as the stent prevents stone impaction. Patency of the prosthesis is therefore not important (bile can flow con-tinuously around the stent), and stent exchanges are typically not required unless the stent migrates spontaneously out of the duct, which may occur when a large sphincterotomy has been performed in an attempt to remove the stone. Need for these long-term endobiliary stents, however, is unusual.

T-Tube Extraction

Extraction of retained common duct stones through a T-tube tract by use of flexible forceps has an 86% success rate. Stones up to 6 and 8 mm in diameter can usually be extracted through 14 and 16 Fr tracts, respectively. Larger stones require crushing, which can often be accomplished by gently pulling the basket with the stone entrapped against the choledochal-sinus tract junction; if not, mechanical intracorporeal lithotripsy can be used. The causes of failure in T-tube extraction include inability to catheterize or re-catheterize the tract, cystic duct stones, and stones truly impacted in the ampulla. The biliary duct can be cleared in one to three sessions in most patients, but 5–15% of patients require more than three sessions. Although complication rates vary between 4% and 5%, death is rare and is typically secondary to complications of severe pancreatitis. The principal disadvantage of this technique is the necessity of leaving the T-tube catheter in place for 5–7 weeks for maturation of the tract to develop prior to removal of the T-tube and cannulation of the tract for stone removal.

Transhepatic Approach

Currently, ERC with or without sphincterotomy is considered the favored approach for most patients with choledocholithiasis; however, when the ERC is unsuccessful in patients in whom the ampulla of Vater may be inaccessible due to previous surgery, percutaneous transhepatic catheterization (PTC) with radiologic interventional techniques is an option. Under fluoroscopic and ultrasonographic guidance, a needle is passed transhepatically into the biliary tree, the bile ducts are opacified with contrast media, and a wire is placed though the needle into the bile duct lumen. The tract is dilated over the guidewire with catheters of increasing size. Depending on the clinical status of the patient and the size and number of stones, a drainage catheter may be placed and time given to allow tract maturation. If the stones are small and the patient is stable, extraction may be attempted during the initial procedure. One series reported a 94% success rate in 54 procedures in 50 patients. Complications occurred in seven patients (13%), and the 30-day mortality was 4% (two patients), including one death from cholangitis and the other from unrelated causes. The complication rate after transhepatic approaches appears greater than those using a T-tube tract; however, comparative controlled trials are lacking. Complications of PTC include bile leak, intraperitoneal bleeding, hemobilia, subcapsular fluid collection, cholangitis, pancreatitis, pneumothorax, and pleural effusions.

Medical Management

Oral bile acids have been used for years to dissolve common duct stones. The success rates, however, are variable, ranging from 10% to 44%. In one randomized, double-blind, placebo-controlled study, 28 patients with uncomplicated, non-obstructing common duct stones were treated with ursodeoxycholic acid (12 mg/kg/d for up to 2 years); the bile duct stones disappeared in 7 of 14 patients in the treatment group and 0 of 14 in the placebo group. Four patients (14%) required operative intervention, including one from the treated and three from the placebo groups. Rowachol (a terpene preparation) is known to further promote stone dissolution. Currently, optimal patient selection, duration of treatment, and optimal dosing has not been determined with these medical treatments of choledocholithiasis. The area in which oral bile acid therapy may play a role is the treatment of asymptomatic patients with small cholesterol duct stones discovered during laparoscopic cholecystectomy. The composition of bile ductal stones may be inferred if cholesterol stones were present in the gallbladder, and small duct stones might dissolve relatively rapidly. Because duct exploration during laparoscopic cholecystectomy might be demanding technically, especially with a small-diameter cystic and/or common bile duct, this dissolution therapy is a reasonable therapeutic alternative; however, this approach needs to be evaluated in clinical trials.

Operative Treatment

By 1990, algorithms for managing duct stones had been well established. Most common duct stones were managed at the time of cholecystectomy, whereas the relatively small number of retained or recurrent duct stones was managed by the interventional radiologist or biliary endoscopists. By the late 1980s, intraoperative cholangiography was a routine part of cholecystectomy, and common duct exploration was performed on the basis of positive findings. Intraoperative cholangiography is a relatively accurate means for diagnosis of duct stones and decreased the frequency of negative results of duct exploration from 65% to 35%. Whether intraoperative cholangiography should be used routinely or selectively at the time of elective cholecystectomy remains controversial. Proponents of routine use of intraoperative cholangiography argue that intraoperative cholangiography decreases the number of negative common duct explorations and detects stones that are not suspected clinically. The prevalence of unsuspected common duct stones is about 2–6%, which favors the use of operative cholangiography in only selected patients. False-positive cholangiograms may result in unnecessary common duct explorations that add morbidity and mortality to cholecystectomy. Hence, if negative results of duct exploration are minimized, the safety of the patient may be enhanced. Because the prevalence of duct stones increases with age, as do the morbidity and mortality from biliary surgery, the mean age of those who undergo common bile duct exploration is older than the mean age of those undergoing simple cholecystectomy. Younger, relatively fit patients have less risk of mortality if common duct exploration is added to cholecystectomy, but this argument does not address the issue of increased morbidity that may accompany duct exploration, such as T-tube complications, bile leaks, and biliary strictures. The frequency of retained common duct stones after common duct exploration, however, can be as high as 10%. The use of routine intraoperative cholangiography after duct exploration to check for missed stones has reduced this figure to about 5%. Intraoperative choledochoscopy may decrease further the incidence of missed choledocholithiasis. The percentage of stones overlooked by cholangiography in which choledochoscopy was used routinely was 13% (88/658), and the overall rate of retained stones was only 2% (11/658).

With the introduction of laparoscopic cholecystectomy, the surgical approach to choledocholithiasis was altered initially, given the lack of equipment and skills for laparoscopic common duct exploration. Currently, these barriers have been overcome in most centers. Preoperative ERCP and stone extraction was recommended in patients in whom common duct stones are suspected (jaundice, increased alkaline phosphatase, CBD dilatation). More recently, however, MRCP or ultrasonography is performed increasingly as a routine preoperative evaluation prior to laparoscopic cholecystectomy in these high-risk patients, and, thus, the indications for preoperative ERCP have become less frequent. Intraoperative cholangiography can be performed easily during laparoscopic cholecystectomy in most patients. Intraoperative cholangiography may detect unsuspected common duct stones in 2–6% patients undergoing laparoscopic cholecystectomy. With training and experience, the common duct can be explored laparoscopically in many of these patients. If the stones are less than five in number and <8 mm in diameter, the common duct can be explored by a small endoscopic choledochoscope (2.7–4 mm diameter) introduced via the cystic duct, called the transcystic approach (Fig. 15.5a). Most patients will require dilatation of the cystic duct. A guide wire is inserted through the cystic duct, and a 5 mm diameter Grunzich balloon is advanced over the guide wire, dilating the cystic duct. The choledochoscope is then introduced via the dilated cystic duct for common duct exploration and stone extraction with appropriately sized baskets. Endoscopic lithotripsy may be used for stones >5mm in diameter. Relative contraindications to the transcystic approach are stones >8 mm, stones proximal to the cystic duct entrance into

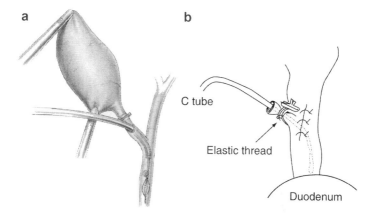

FIGURE 15.5. (**a**) Transcystic approach. The lumen of the cystic duct is dilated up to 5 mm with a balloon. An endoscope can be introduced into the common duct to retrieve stones. (**b**) Primary closure. When a choledochotomy is made for duct exploration and stone removal, the choledochotomy can be reapproximated by suture close with or without a transcystic decompressive tube choledochoscopy. It can also be primarily suture-closed with or without placing a C-tube for biliary decompression.

the common duct, a small friable cystic duct, and ten or more stones. In some reports, the transcystic approach is applicable in about 85% of patients with a success rate of about 90%. When successful, it is also more cost-effective than postoperative endoscopic sphincterotomy and duct clearance.

When the transcystic approach is either contraindicated or technically impossible, common duct exploration may be carried out via a laparoscopic choledochotomy with use of a biliary endoscope for ductal clearance of stones. This approach, however, requires more advanced laparoscopic skills. T-tubes are used in patients in whom there is concern for possible retained debris or stones, distal ductal spasm, pancreatitis, or general poor tissue quality secondary to malnutrition or infection. In one series of 57 patients, a T-tube was placed in 38 patients (67%), while primary closure without a T-tube was carried out in 19 (33%) (Fig. 15.5b). There were no serious complications in the group of patients who underwent choledochotomy and primary ductal closure with or without T-tube placement. Placement of a small-diameter (16 Fr) tube via the cystic duct stump may be of value for decompression and postoperative cholangiography when the choledochotomy is to be reapproximated by suture closure.

Because the pathogenesis of recurrent duct stones involves stasis and/or relative obstruction in most cases, surgical dictum suggests the addition of a drainage procedure (sphincterotomy, choledochoduodenostomy, or choledochojejunostomy) to duct exploration. These additional drainage procedures are not required as part of the initial duct exploration unless the duct stones are primary, or when complete clearance of multiple stones is in doubt, a stone is impacted in the distal common bile duct in an elderly and frail patient, or the distal bile duct is obstructed by ampullary stenosis or chronic pancreatitis. In the setting of primary common duct stones, which almost always is associated with ductal dilation, even in the absence of a true, distal, mechanical obstruction, most surgeons would advocate one of these drainage procedures. The need for a drainage procedure for "recurrent" choledocholithiasis has been the subject of a prospective, randomized study. No patient who underwent choledochoduodenostomy required subsequent reoperation for recurrent biliary tract disease, whereas 13% of those who underwent sphincteroplasty and 23% of those who had T-tube drainage alone required reoperation for recurrent stone disease. With the ability of endoscopic sphincterotomy, a choledochoduodenostomy is preferred in patients with a long stenosis from chronic pancreatitis or if the surgeon has difficulty accessing the papilla. If the common duct exceeds 15 mm in diameter, biliary stasis (either functional or mechanical) is highly suspect, and a choledochoduodenostomy is recommended.

Acute Suppurative Cholangitis

Endoscopic sphincterotomy is considered the procedure of choice in patients with acute cholangitis. Experience was reported with urgent (mean of 1.5 days after admission) endoscopic drainage of the biliary tree in 105 patients with acute calculous cholangitis who did not respond to conservative management. Drainage was successful in 97% of patients, with resolution of fever, abdominal pain, and abnormal liver tests. Among those with hemodynamic instability, 2 of 4 patients, compared with 3 (8%) of 38 patients, died who underwent endoscopic drainage within 72 h of diagnosis or >72 h, respectively. No death occurred in patients without hemodynamic instability, regardless of the timing of drainage. A retrospective review of patients with acute cholangitis due to choledocholithiasis treated with operative drainage versus endoscopic sphincterotomy found a lesser mortality after sphincterotomy (5% vs. 21%). Similarly, a randomized, prospective study comparing the outcome of endoscopic drainage ($n = 41$) with surgical decompression ($n = 41$) in patients with acute cholangitis due to choledocholithiasis identified a markedly less morbidity and mortality in the patients treated endoscopically.

Selected Readings

Haws RH, Sherman S (2001) Choledocholithiasis. In: Haubrich WS, Schaffner F, Berk JE (eds), Bockus Gastro-enterology, Chapter 142, 5th edn., vol. 3. W.B. Saunders, Philadelphia, pp. 2745–2789

Joyce WP, Keane R, Burke GJ, et al. (1991) Identification of bile duct stones in patients undergoing laparoscopic cholecystectomy. Br J Surg 78:1174–1176

Kats J, Kraai M, Dijkstra AJ, et al. (2003) Magnetic resonance cholangiopancreaticography as a diagnostic tool for common bile duct stones: a comparison with ERCP and clinical follow-up. Dig Surg 20:32–37

Lezoche E, Paganini AM (2000) Technical considerations and laparoscopic bile duct exploration: transcystic and choledochotomy. Semin Laparosc Surg 7:262–278

Martin DJ, Vernon DR, Toouli J (2006) Surgical versus endoscopic treatment of bile duct stones. Cochrane Database Syst Rev 19: CD003327

NIH state-of-the-science statement on endoscopic retrograde cholangiopancreatography (ERCP) for diagnosis and therapy. NIH Consens State Sci Statements 19:1–26

Petelin JB (2003) Laparoscopic common bile duct exploration. Surg Endosc 17:1705–1715

Tokumura H, Umezawa A, Cao H, et al. (2002) Laparoscopic management of common bile duct stones: trans-cystic approach and choledochotomy. J Hepatobiliary Pancreat Surg 9:206–212

16
Choledochal Cysts

Chi-Leung Liu

Pearls and Pitfalls

- Five types of choledochal cysts are recognized according to the Todani classification system, which can be further classified into eight alphanumeric subtypes.
- Sixty percent present in the first decade of life.
- Cystoduodenostomy or cystojejunostomy results in a high incidence of long-term complications including anastomotic stricture, cholangitis, biliary calculi, and biliary tract malignancy.
- Total excision with Roux-en-Y hepaticojejunostomy is the treatment of choice.
- Hepatic resection is required in selected cases with intrahepatic extension.
- Liver transplantation is indicated for type V choledochal cyst (Caroli's disease).

Introduction

Choledochal cyst is an uncommon anomaly and is estimated to occur in between 1 in 13,000 to 1 in 2 million live births. It is more common in Asian populations and in females. Initially described in 1852, choledochal cysts were classified into three types by Alonso-Lej et al. in 1959: *type I*, a solitary fusiform

K.I. Bland et al. (eds.), *Liver and Biliary Surgery*,
DOI 10.1007/978-1-84996-429-6_16,
© Springer-Verlag London Limited 2011

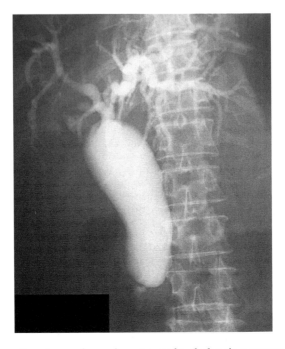

FIGURE 16.1. An endoscopic retrograde cholangiopancreatogram (ERCP) film showing a fusiform type (type 1) choledochal cyst.

extrahepatic cyst (80%; Fig. 16.1); *type II*, a supraduodenal saccular cyst draining into the extrahepatic bile duct (5%); *type III*, an intraduodenal diverticulum (choledochocele, 5%). *Type IV* (multiple extrahepatic cysts with or without intrahepatic cysts, 10%) and *type V* (multiple small intrahepatic cysts, Caroli's disease, <1%) were added to this classification by Todani et al. in 1977. More than 3,300 cases of choledochal cysts have been reported in the literature, and more than half were reported by Japanese investigators. The diagnosis of choledochal cysts is usually made in the first few years of life; more than 60% of all affected patients are diagnosed in the first decade. Presentation in adulthood is uncommon and is often associated with complication of the cyst.

Etiology

The "long common channel theory" proposed by Babbitt et al. is most widely accepted. The disease is thought to be a result of anomalous junction of the common bile duct with the pancreatic duct (anomalous pancreatobiliary junction [APBJ]). An APBJ is characterized when the pancreatic duct enters the common bile duct 1 cm or more proximal to where the common bile duct reaches the Ampulla of Vater. Miyano and Yamataka have demonstrated such APBJs in more than 90% of their patients with choledochal cysts. The APBJ allows pancreatic secretions and enzymes to reflux into the common bile duct. In the relatively alkaline conditions found in the common bile duct, pancreatic proenzymes can be activated, resulting in inflammation and weakening of the bile duct wall. Severe damage leads to complete denuding of the common bile duct mucosa. In addition, defects in epithelialization and recanalization of the developing bile ducts during organogenesis and congenital weakness of the duct wall have also been implicated. However, this theory cannot satisfactorily explain the etiology of diverticular choledochal cysts, choledochocele, or intrahepatic cyst formation.

Presentation and Investigation

Choledochal cysts can present at any age. With the increasing use of imaging studies in clinical management, more cases are diagnosed incidentally. Neonates or children usually present with the triad of abdominal pain, abdominal mass, and jaundice; in previous reviews the triad was present in only 38% of the patients. Initial manifestation in adults is rare, and the clinical presentation is usually nonspecific right upper quadrant abdominal pain, jaundice, acute cholangitis, or acute pancreatitis. Hence, endoscopic retrograde cholangiopancreatogram (ERCP) is one of the most commonly used methods for diagnosis of choledochal cysts, especially in the initial management of acute cholangitis, acute pancreatitis, and biliary malignancies. Other investigative tools for patients with choledochal cysts include ultrasonography, radionuclide scanning, computed tomography (CT), and magnetic resonance imaging (MRI) cholangiography.

Complications of these cysts include liver abscess, cirrhosis, and portal hypertension. The pathogenic mechanism of bile reflux into the pancreatic duct related to the APBJ lesion is associated with choledochal cyst and may result in recurrent acute pancreatitis. Pregnancy can precipitate or worsen complications, especially spontaneous rupture of the choledochal cyst. Carcinomas of the biliary tract, including cholangiocarcinoma and carcinoma of the gallbladder (Fig. 16.2) are well-recognized complications and portend a poor prognosis because of the difficulty of early diagnosis. Carcinoma has been reported to occur in 2.5–28% of patients with choledochal cysts, representing a risk at least 20 times greater than that of the general population. The risk is age-related and reported to be 14.5% in patients 20 years of age. Possible factors for carcinogenesis in choledochal cysts include chronic inflammation, bile stagnation with possible development of

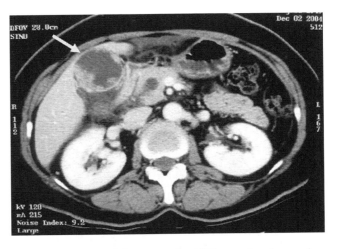

FIGURE 16.2. A computed tomography (CT) scan showing carcinoma of the gallbladder (arrow) complicating choledochal cyst.

carcinogens, and a spare distribution of the protective mucin-secreting glands of the bile duct.

Biliary tract malignancy complicating choledochal cysts is reportedly enhanced by cystenterostomy. It is postulated that pancreatic juice easily regurgitates into the bile duct through an anomalous junction of the pancreatobiliary ductal system in patients with choledochal cysts, and enteric drainage causes pancreatic juice in the cyst to become activated due to the influx of enteric content. Therefore, inflammatory changes of the cysts are accelerated and initiate carcinoma. The mean age at detection of malignancy complicating choledochal cysts is influenced by previous internal drainage operations. Biliary tract malignancy in patients with internal drainage was found to occur 15 years earlier than those without a previous drainage procedure; most cases of malignant degeneration were detected, on average, 10 years after an internal drainage procedure. Since carcinoma that develops from choledochal cysts has a very dismal prognosis, even radical surgical excision is often noncurative. Most patients die within 2 years of the diagnosis. Excision biliary reconstruction, rather than internal drainage, are recommended as the treatment of choice for choledochal cysts.

Treatment

Early reports suggest that drainage operations including cystoduodenostomy, or cystojejunostomy without excision of the cyst, result in satisfactory outcomes in the treatment of choledochal cysts. However, it has become evident that 30–50% of patients with cystoduodenostomy had late complications, such as anastomotic stricture, cholangitis, secondary biliary cirrhosis, biliary calculi, and biliary tract malignancy. Although Roux-en-Y cystojejunostomy was developed to avoid reflux of the duodenal contents into the biliary tree, acute cholangitis and other problems still commonly occur. While cystenterostomy is technically easier, cyst excision with Roux-en-Y hepaticojejunostomy can be performed with low morbidity and mortality, and should be the treatment of choice for the disease. With increased risk of developing malignancy of the biliary tract and the potential for poor outcomes in patients with choledochal cysts, resection of the cysts should be recommended when diagnosed, even in the asymptomatic patient. Complete excision of the cyst is emphasized to avoid malignant transformation in the cystic remnant.

Although the accepted treatment of choledochal cyst is essentially surgical, irrespective of the age of the patient, long-term management of patients with Caroli's disease remains controversial. In addition to surgical treatment, bile stasis can be prevented by internal drainage via ERCP with endoscopic sphincterotomy, biliary stent placement, and stone extraction, together with administration of ursodeoxycholic acid. Endoscopic treatment is also the method of choice for uncomplicated choledochocele (type III), after which long-term follow-up is probably unnecessary. However, carcinoma may rarely coexist with choledochocele, and other measures, such as endoscopic ultrasonography and biopsy, may be required to exclude malignancy.

Caroli's disease, Todani's type V choledochal cyst, is a rare congenital disorder characterized by multifocal segmental and cystic dilations of the intrahepatic bile ducts. Whether conservative or surgical treatment is preferred remains controversial. Clinical presentation of Caroli's patients range from totally asymptomatic for many years to cholangitis, intrahepatic abscesses, hepatolithiasis, or jaundice. The rate of malignant transformation to cholangiocarcinoma has been estimated to be 7%, or about 100 times greater than that of the general population. In patients with Caroli's disease confined to one lobe, hemihepatectomy has been advocated for surgical treatment. This aggressive surgical approach has been associated with low operative morbidity and mortality. On the contrary, patients with diffuse Caroli's disease involving both lobes of the liver are difficult to manage. Despite advances in medical and endoscopic treatment, non-surgical treatment fails to result in permanent recovery from symptoms of the disease. For patients with diffuse hepatic fibrosis, hepatolithiasis with repeated cholangitis, and secondary biliary cirrhosis, liver transplantation using grafts from deceased or live donors has been reported with satisfactory survival outcomes.

Selected Readings

Babbitt DP, Starshak RJ, Clemett AR (1973) Choledochal cyst: a concept of etiology. Am J Roentgenol Radium Ther Nucl Med 119:57–62

Ishida M, Tsuchida Y, Saito S, et al. (1970) Primary excision of choledochal cysts. Surgery 68:884–888

Kasai M, Asakura Y, Taira Y (1970) Surgical treatment of choledochal cyst. Ann Surg 172:844–851

Liu CL, Fan ST, Lo CM, et al. (1997) Choledochal cysts in adults. Arch Surg 137:465–468

Miyano T, Yamataka A (1997) Choledochal cysts. Curr Opin Pediatr 9:283–288

Nagata E, Sakai K, Kinoshita H, et al. (1986) Choledochal cyst: complications of anomalous connection between the choledochus and pancreatic duct and carcinoma of the biliary tract. World J Surg 10:102–110

O'Neill Jr JA, Templeton Jr JM, Schnaufer L, et al. (1987) Recent experience with choledochal cyst. Ann Surg 205:533–540

Rossi RL, Silverman ML, Braasch JW, et al. (1987) Carcinomas arising in cystic conditions of the bile ducts. A clinical and pathologic study. Ann Surg 205:377–384

Todani T, Watanabe Y, Toki A, et al. (2003) Classification of congenital biliary cystic disease: special reference to type Ic and IVA cysts with primary ductal stricture. J Hepato-biliary Pancreat Surg 10:340–344

Voyles CR, Smadja C, Shands WC, et al. (1983) Carcinoma in choledochal cysts. Age-related incidence. Arch Surg 118:986–988

17
Biliary Dyskinesia: Functional Gallbladder and Sphincter of Oddi Disorders

Cary B. Aarons, Arthur F. Stucchi, and James M. Becker

Pearls and Pitfalls

- The sphincter of Oddi, which surrounds the confluence of the distal common bile duct and pancreatic ducts is composed of three sphincters: a biliary sphincter (*sphincter choledochus*), a pancreatic sphincter (*sphincter pancreaticus*), and an ampullary sphincter (*sphincter ampullae*).
- Laparoscopic cholecystectomy is the primary treatment for patients with gallbladder dysmotility.
- Biliary pain after cholecystectomy, in the absence of retained stones, is due typically to sphincter of Oddi dysfunction (SOD).
- Biliary ultrasonography and hepatobiliary scintigraphy have low sensitivity and specificity in diagnosing SOD compared to sphincter of Oddi manometry.
- Sphincter of Oddi manometry (SOM) is associated with high rates of post-ERCP pancreatitis.
- Endoscopic sphincterotomy is the treatment of choice in patients with type I biliary SOD.
- In patients with type III biliary SOD, the response to endoscopic sphincterotomy is generally poor. Thorough evaluation in these patients is crucial.

K.I. Bland et al. (eds.), *Liver and Biliary Surgery*,
DOI 10.1007/978-1-84996-429-6_17,
© Springer-Verlag London Limited 2011

Introduction

Surgeons are consulted frequently to evaluate patients presenting with epigastric pain of unknown origin. In some cases, these patients may have already undergone non-invasive imaging studies that have failed to identify the origin of their complaints. Often times, these patients have had recurrent episodes of this pain severe enough to interrupt daily activities or lead to an emergency room visit. When an obvious anatomic or physiologic abnormality or disease cannot be identified, the diagnosis is labeled invariably as a functional gastrointestinal disorder. This somewhat vague diagnosis can be problematic for the patient and the surgeon, because there is no rational basis for an effective treatment plan. Recognizing that functional gastrointestinal disorders have been so poorly understood for decades, a panel of experts at the International Congress of Gastroenterology in 1988 subsequently wrote the first consensus paper on functional gastrointestinal disorders. A committee was then established to develop a classification system for all 21 "functional" gastrointestinal disorders. This first report in 1990 was the beginning of the Rome Foundation's Rome Criteria process and set the stage for organizing study groups composed of internationally recognized investigators who have legitimized the functional gastrointestinal disorders which include biliary dyskinesia or functional gallbladder and sphincter of Oddi disorders.

In late 2006, the Rome Foundation released the new Rome III criteria on functional gastrointestinal disorders that proposed a substantial paradigm shift for diagnosing and treating functional biliary disorders. The term "biliary dyskinesia" describes a group of complex functional biliary disorders in patients with symptoms indicative of biliary tract disease without definable structural abnormalities such as gallstones. To establish more symptom-based diagnostic criteria for functional gastrointestinal disorders, experts proposed to no longer group together the functional biliary disorders. Instead, each disorder is now classified according to the anatomic site of the suspected dysmotility disorder. Based on

TABLE 17.1. Rome III classifications for functional gallbladder and sphincter of Oddi disorders (Reprinted from Behar J et al., 2006b. Copyright 2006. With permission from American Gastroenterological Association).

Functional gallbladder disorder
Functional biliary sphincter of Oddi disorder
Functional pancreatic sphincter of Oddi disorder

expert consensus, new clinical criteria have been proposed for the diagnosis of functional gallbladder and sphincter of Oddi disorders. Three subsets of biliary dysmotility disorders are now recognized: functional gallbladder disorder; functional biliary sphincter of Oddi disorder; and, functional pancreatic sphincter of Oddi disorder (Table 17.1).

Functional Gallbladder and Sphincter of Oddi Disorders

The regulation of secretions from the liver, gallbladder, and pancreas into the duodenum is physiologically complex. As discussed below, integrated actions of multiple sphincters regulate this flow, and any disruption may lead to intermittent upper abdominal pain, transient increases in serum liver or pancreatic enzymes, common bile duct dilatation, or episodes of pancreatitis. Dysmotility disorders of the gallbladder and sphincter of Oddi are relatively uncommon. About 30% of the three-quarters of a million cholecystectomies performed in the United States annually are for a functional biliary disorder. Many terms have been used to describe functional biliary disorders, including biliary dyskinesia, chronic acalculous cholecystitis, gallbladder or bile duct dyskinesia, biliary spasm, papillary stenosis, postcholecystectomy syndrome, and sphincter of Oddi dysfunction; however, these functional disorders are best characterized by symptoms arising from pathology of the gallbladder or the sphincter of Oddi.

The consensus-based guidelines recommend that patients with epigastric or upper right quadrant pain who do not meet the Rome III symptom-based criteria should not undergo any invasive diagnostic procedures such as endoscopic retrograde cholangiopancreatography (ERCP). Instead, patients who meet the criteria should be assessed initially with noninvasive procedures and eventually with therapeutic trials that will more likely identify the majority of patients whose pain is not biliary or pancreatic in origin and will therefore not require further diagnostic investigation. Before discussing the diagnostic algorithms and treatment options, an overview of the basic anatomy of the sphincter of Oddi will familiarize the reader with the intricate anatomic relationship of the sphincteric muscles with the convergence of bile duct and the pancreatic duct at the duodenal wall.

Anatomy and Regulation of the Sphincter of Oddi

The sphincter of Oddi is a muscular structure that encompasses the confluence of the distal common bile duct and the pancreatic duct as they pass through the wall of the duodenum. The sphincter is composed of small circular and longitudinal muscular segments 6–10 mm in length contained primarily within the wall of the duodenum (Fig. 17.1). A circular collection of muscle fibers, known as the *sphincter choledochus*, or the sphincter of the common bile duct, encircles the duodenal segment of the common bile duct and the ampulla of Vater and maintains resistance to bile flow during fasting, permitting the gallbladder to fill and preventing the reflux of duodenal content. At its convergence with the bile duct, the distal pancreatic duct is also encircled by a circular muscular structure, the *sphincter pancreaticus*, or sphincter of the pancreatic duct, which is interconnected with the muscles of the *sphincter choledochus* in a figure-eight pattern. The motility of the sphincter of Oddi is complex, and because the bile and pancreatic ductal sphincters

Sphincer of oddi complex

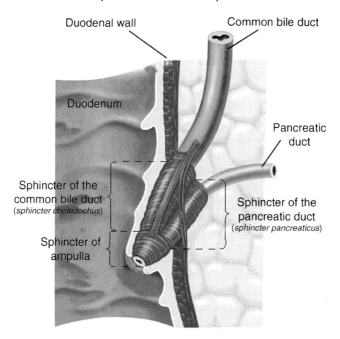

FIGURE 17.1. Anatomy of the sphincter of Oddi complex. The sphincter of Oddi is a complex of three individual sphincters: (a) the muscle fibers of the sphincter of Oddi surround the intraduodenal segment of the common bile duct and the ampulla of Vater; (b) a circular aggregate of muscle fibers surround the choledochus; and (c) a separate structure, called the sphincter pancreaticus, encircles the distal pancreatic duct. The muscle fibers of the sphincter pancreaticus are interlocked with those of the sphincter choledochus in a figure eight pattern. The sphincter of ampulla lies at the convergence of the biliary and pancreatic sphincters (Adapted from Boyden, 1957, and reproduced from, Rass BD, 2006. With permission of UpToDate).

function independently, the Rome III criteria classifies their dysmotility disorders separately (Table 17.1).

The regulation of the sphincter of Oddi varies in the fasting and fed states. The gallbladder contracts secondary to neurohormonal stimuli, and its function in regulating bile flow from the liver is related closely to sphincter of Oddi function. During fasting, flow of bile from the gallbladder occurs in concert with the contractile activity in the stomach and duodenum. After a meal, cholecystokinin (CCK), which is released from the duodenum, is the main stimulus for gallbladder contraction and sphincter of Oddi relaxation. A variety of medications also affect sphincter of Oddi tone, including nitrates, calcium channel blockers, and narcotics.

The underlying pathology of functional biliary disorders stems from uncoordinated contractions between the gallbladder and the sphincter of Oddi during CCK stimulation. The resulting gallbladder distension causes acute inflammation and dysmotility; however, fibrosis and chronic inflammation have also been implicated in dysmotility. Pathologic examination of the gallbladder in patients with biliary dysmotility generally reveals either chronic cholecystitis, cholesterolosis, or even normal histology.

Diagnostic Criteria for Functional Gallbladder and Sphincter of Oddi Disorders

The new Rome III classification is based on the assertion that patients with functional disorders of the gallbladder and sphincter of Oddi present with clusters of similar symptoms. Based on symptom-based diagnostic algorithms, the new criteria are more restrictive in an effort to avoid unnecessary invasive biliary and pancreatic procedures. Biliary dyskinesia is now divided into functional motility disorders of the gallbladder, biliary sphincter of Oddi, and pancreatic sphincter of Oddi; each has a specific diagnostic algorithm and treatment plan. Treatment strategies are aimed at the specific anatomic site of the suspected dysfunction. These functional disorders present with epigastric and right upper quadrant pain and symptoms not easily distinguished from unrelated functional gastrointestinal disorders such as gastroesophageal reflux, irritable bowel, dyspepsia, and cholelithiasis. Sphincter of Oddi dysfunction can cause liver and pancreatic abnormalities; thus, these disorders must also be excluded before patients suspected of having biliary dyskinesia undergo invasive diagnostic procedures or operation.

Patients presenting with biliary-type pain must experience *all* of the following symptoms: recurrent episodes of epigastric or right upper quadrant pain that persist for 30 min or longer and occur at different intervals, usually not daily. The pain generally builds to a steady, non-colicky level and is severe enough to interrupt normal activities or lead to an emergency room visit (Table 17.2). Severe episodes may be associated with nausea and vomiting and pain radiating to the back and/or right infrasubscapular region.

TABLE 17.2. Rome III diagnostic criteria for functional gallbladder and sphincter of Oddi disorders (Reprinted from Behar J et al., 2006a. With permission by the Rome Foundation).

Must include episodes of pain located in the epigastrium and/or right upper quadrant and *all* of the following symptoms:

1. Episodes lasting 30 min or longer

2. Recurrent symptoms occurring at different intervals (not daily)

3. The pain builds up to a steady level

4. The pain is moderate to severe enough to interrupt the patient's daily activities or lead to an emergency department visit

5. The pain is not relieved by bowel movements

6. The pain is not relieved by postural change

7. The pain is not relieved by antacids

8. Exclusion of other structural disease that would explain the symptoms

Supportive criteria

The pain may present with one or more of the following:

1. Associated nausea and vomiting

2. Radiates to the back and/or right subscapular region

3. Awakens from sleep in the middle of the night

Functional Gallbladder Disorder

Although the prevalence of gallbladder dysmotility in the absence of lithogenic bile is not known, population-based studies suggest the occurrence of biliary pain in patients with a negative gallbladder ultrasonography of about 8% in males to 20% in females. By definition, patients with gallbladder dysfunction have impaired gallbladder emptying. Gallbladder dysfunction is characterized by a motility defect that stems initially from either a metabolic disorder such as cholesterol supersaturated bile or a primary dysmotility of the gallbladder in the absence of alterations in bile composition. Either scenario leads to a functional obstruction in the cystic duct, leading to an increase in gallbladder pressure. The associated inflammation often amplifies sensory firing and exacerbates the condition.

Clinical Presentation

The symptoms manifest with biliary-type pain. These symptoms may occur concurrently in the setting of low-grade, chronic abdominal pain. Although gallbladder dysmotility is often referred to as chronic acalculous cholecystitis or cystic duct syndrome, gallbladder dysmotility refers to the subset of patients with biliary pain stemming from intrinsic gallbladder muscle dysfunction or the development of dysfunction due to chronic cholecystitis. Patients must fulfill all of the diagnostic criteria for functional gallbladder and sphincter of Oddi disorders in Table 17.2 with the addition of those criteria for functional gallbladder disorder as well (Table 17.3).

Diagnostic evaluation: The Rome III guidelines propose the following criteria: (1) absence of gallstones, biliary sludge, or microlithiasis; (2) a gallbladder ejection fraction of less than 40%; and (3) a positive response with absence of the pain for >12 months after cholecystectomy. The algorithm for the diagnostic work-up is shown in Fig. 17.2. The most fundamental step is a thorough history and physical examination to exclude another functional gastrointestinal disorder. Tests of liver

TABLE 17.3. Diagnostic criteria for functional gallbladder disorder (Reprinted from Behar J et al., 2006a. With permission by the Rome Foundation).

Must include all of the following:

1. Criteria for functional gallbladder and sphincter of Oddi disorder in Table 17.2

2. Gallbladder is present

3. Normal liver enzymes, conjugated bilirubin, and amylase/lipase

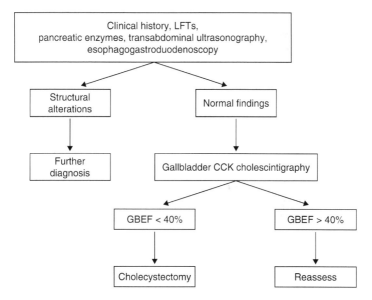

FIGURE 17.2. Algorithm of the diagnostic work-up and management of functional gallbladder disorders. Abbreviations: LFTs = liver function tests; CCK = cholecystokinin; GBEF = gallbladder ejection fraction (Reprinted from Behar J et al., 2006a. With permission by the Rome Foundation).

biochemistries and pancreatic enzymes should be obtained to rule out other possible diagnoses. These tests are normal in the presence of gallbladder motor dysfunction.

A transabdominal ultrasonography of the upper abdomen is essential. The biliary tract and pancreas appear normal without gallstones or sludge. If microlithiasis (stones <3 mm) or sludge within the biliary tract are suspected, endoscopic ultrasonography (EUS) is particularly useful due to its increased sensitivity. An upper gastrointestinal endoscopy is indicated to exclude significant abnormalities of the esophagus, stomach, and duodenum and to support the diagnosis of a functional gallbladder disorder.

If the above testing is normal, evaluation of gallbladder motor function is indicated. Assuming the cystic duct is patent, gallbladder emptying is assessed by quantitative CCK-stimulated cholescintigraphy using technetium 99m-labeled hepatobiliary iminodiacetic acid (HIDA) analogs. These compounds are readily excreted into the bile and are concentrated in the gallbladder. A low gallbladder ejection fraction after CCK administration is a good indicator of impaired gallbladder motor function and primary gallbladder dysfunction. Decreased gallbladder emptying can arise from impaired gallbladder contraction or increased resistance of the sphincter of Oddi. Diabetes and drugs such as calcium channel blockers can impair gallbladder emptying and need to be considered. A gallbladder ejection fraction of <40% is considered abnormal and suggestive of a functional disorder. Ultrasonography and cholescintigraphy have increased sensitivity and specificity, but false positives and false negatives occur in the setting of severe liver disease, previous sphincterotomy, and patients receiving total parenteral nutrition.

Patients that meet the symptom-based criteria but have gallbladder ejection fractions pose a more difficult diagnostic scenario. Additional work-up to exclude other structural abnormalities by computed tomography may be warranted. A small number may benefit from diet modification, but if symptoms persist for 4–6 months, then laparoscopic cholecystectomy may be indicated.

Treatment and outcome: Once the diagnosis of functional gallbladder disorder is confirmed, the only treatment option is cholecystectomy. Several randomized studies have shown that about 90% of patients undergoing a cholecystectomy experience resolution of symptoms.

Functional Biliary Sphincter of Oddi Disorder

The sphincter of Oddi, located anatomically at the duodenal junction of the biliary and pancreatic ducts, plays a key role in the regulation of secretions (Fig. 17.1). During digestion, contractions of the sphincter of Oddi create resistance and backpressure in the bile duct which triggers a reflex that relaxes the gallbladder. Sphincter of Oddi dysfunction has been defined as a motility disorder characterized primarily by symptoms of pancreaticobiliary obstruction in the absence of either structural or organic disease. Sphincter of Oddi dysfunction can involve abnormalities in the biliary sphincter, pancreatic sphincter, or both. The new Rome III criteria classify these into two separate functional disorders. Although patients with an intact gallbladder can present with symptoms of a functional disorder of the biliary sphincter of Oddi, most clinical information regarding this disorder has been gained from postcholecystectomy patients.

Until recently, patients presenting with symptoms of biliary sphincter of Oddi dysfunction after cholecystectomy have been categorized subjectively according to their clinical presentation and test findings. The Rome III classification system is more clinically applicable to avoid the need for unnecessary invasive procedures such as ERCP. Contrast drainage times are not required and noninvasive methods such as ultrasonography should be used to measure the common bile duct diameter.

The majority of patients present with the biliary type, most commonly after cholecystectomy. While about 20% of patients have pain after cholecystectomy, only 1–2% will be associated with biliary sphincter of Oddi dysfunction, and it is more common in females.

Clinical presentation: Biliary sphincter of Oddi dysfunction is characterized by motility abnormalities of the sphincter of Oddi associated with biliary pain. Patients presenting with episodes of biliary pain will often have transient elevations in serum transaminases, alkaline phosphatase, or conjugated bilirubin levels indicative of a temporary biliary tract

TABLE 17.4. Diagnostic criteria for functional biliary sphincter of Oddi disorder (Reprinted from Behar J et al., 2006a. With permission by the Rome Foundation).

Must include all of the following:

1. Criteria for functional gallbladder and sphincter of Oddi disorder in Table 17.2

2. Normal amylase/lipase

Supportive criteria

Increased serum transaminases, alkaline phosphatase, or conjugated bilirubin temporally related to at least two pain episodes

obstruction (Table 17.4). Indicators of pancreatic sphincter of Oddi dysmotility such as serum levels of amylase/lipase are normal. The similarities in the presenting clinical symptoms between biliary sphincter of Oddi and gallbladder dysfunction can make the diagnosis difficult, but because most patients have already had a cholecystectomy, the diagnosis of biliary sphincter of Oddi dysfunction is usually made after cholecystectomy.

Biliary sphincter of Oddi dysfunction is described in two categories: sphincter of Oddi stenosis and sphincter of Oddi dysmotility or dyskinesia. Sphincter of Oddi stenosis is an anatomic abnormality due to inflammation or scarring, which occurs after passage of a gallstone. In contrast, sphincter of Oddi dyskinesia is a functional abnormality due to spasm of the sphincter. Alone, biliary pain is an unreliable clinical tool to classify biliary sphincter of Oddi dysfunction; therefore, more objective clinical criteria are necessary to classify biliary sphincter of Oddi dysfunction into three subsets. Patients that present with biliary-type pain, increases in transaminases, bilirubin, or alkaline phosphatase of at least two-fold on two or more occasions concurrently with a common bile duct >8 mm on ultrasonography are classified as type I (Table 17.5). About two-thirds of biliary type I patients have stenosis of the sphincter of Oddi. Type II patients present with biliary-type pain but only one of the previously mentioned laboratory or imaging abnormalities. Just over half of

TABLE 17.5. Milwaukee classification of biliary sphincter of Oddi dysfunction (Reprinted from Behar J et al., 2006a. With permission by the Rome Foundation).

Type I (biliary stenosis)
Moderate to severe biliary pain
Transient increases in ALT, AST, alkaline phosphatase > 2 times normal values, or conjugated bilirubin documented on two or more occasions
Dilated common bile duct (>12 mm)
Delayed drainage of ERCP contrast (>45 min)
Type II (biliary dyskinesia)
Biliary pain and one or two of the following:
Abnormal liver function tests (>2 times normal)
Dilated common bile duct (>8 mm at ultrasonography)
Delayed drainage of ERCP contrast (>45 min)
Type III (biliary dyskinesia)
Biliary pain only and none of the above criteria

these type II patients have abnormal manometry studies indicative of biliary sphincter of Oddi dysfunction. In type III patients, less than half have manometric evidence of biliary sphincter of Oddi dysfunction, and their primary complaint is recurrent biliary-type pain without abnormalities in laboratory values or imaging.

Diagnostic evaluation: The algorithm for the diagnostic work-up of patients with suspected biliary sphincter of Oddi dysfunction is shown in Fig. 17.3 and is utilized primarily in patients who have undergone a cholecystectomy. Gallbladder dysfunction must first be ruled out in patients with gallbladder *in situ*. The Rome III guidelines propose that the initial work-up should begin with liver biochemistries and pancreatic enzymes performed shortly after an episode. Depending on symptoms, potential structural causes should be eliminated carefully using the least invasive imaging techniques, such as transabdominal or endoscopic ultrasonography, CT,

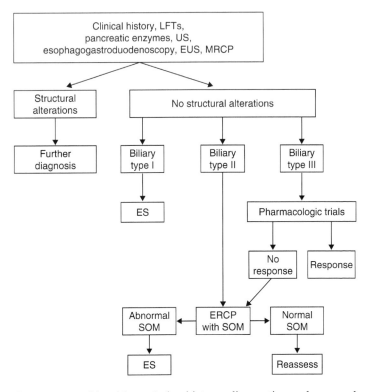

FIGURE 17.3. Algorithm of the history, diagnostic work-up, and treatment of patients suspected with functional biliary SO disorder with types 1, 2 and 3. ERCP = endoscopic retrograde cholangiopancreatography; ES = endoscopic sphincterotomy; EUS = endoscopic ultrasonography; LFT = liver function test; MRCP = magnetic resonance cholangiopancreatography; SOM = sphincter of Oddi manometry; US = ultrasonography (Reprinted from Behar J et al., 2006a. With permission by the Rome Foundation).

and magnetic resonance cholangiography (MRCP). Patients with biliary type I sphincter of Oddi dysfunction may undergo endoscopic sphincterotomy without further diagnostic testing such as sphincter of Oddi manometry. Sphincter of Oddi manometry is recommended in patients with suspected biliary type II and, if strongly suspected, in type III sphincter of Oddi dysfunction. Invasive procedures such as ERCP should be avoided unless a thorough clinical evaluation has concluded that potential benefits exceed the risks. If noninvasive imaging has not detected structural alterations and the pain is disabling despite therapeutic trials with proton pump inhibitors and spasmolytics, then ERCP is indicated. ERCP offers the ability to utilize sphincter of Oddi manometry, the most effective test for defining objectively the motility of the biliary sphincter. A pressure sensor is passed across the sphincter to record basal resting pressure and phasic contractions. Normal basal sphincter pressure is <40 mmHg, and phasic contractions are predominantly antegrade. In sphincter of Oddi stenosis, the basal pressure is increased, while in biliary sphincter of Oddi dysmotility, the sphincter has rapid phasic contractions, excessive retrograde contractions, or increased contractions with CCK injection instead of the normal relaxation. Although sphincter of Oddi manometry is a technically demanding, invasive procedure associated with a 30% risk of post-ERCP pancreatitis, it is superior to hepatobiliary scintigraphy and fatty meal ultrasonography, that cannot accurately differentiate the three types of sphincter of Oddi dysfunction.

Treatment and outcome: The therapeutic paradigm is aimed at reducing the resistance to flow of bile caused by a stenotic or dysfunctional biliary sphincter. Medical therapy with nitroglycerine, the calcium channel blocker nifedipine, and botulinum toxin (Botox) injections into the sphincter have been shown to reduce sphincter pressure and improve bile flow. Medical therapy may be an attractive initial approach, but there are no long-term studies on the outcome. Botox injections directly into the sphincter may serve as a diagnostic tool for biliary sphincter of Oddi dysfunction and as a predictor of outcome after sphincterotomy. Because most medical therapies are not effective or long-lasting, the treatment of choice is sphincterotomy. Division of the sphincter can be accomplished by an endoscopic or transduodenal approach; however, endoscopic sphincterotomy is the most widely used therapeutic procedure especially for patients with type I biliary sphincter of Oddi dysfunction (biliary stenosis), because it is less expensive, cosmetically more acceptable, and has a lower morbidity than open surgery. Management of type II biliary sphincter of Oddi dysfunction is more complex and requires coordinated discussion among the patient, the surgeon, and the gastroenterologist. A significant proportion of patients with suspected type II sphincter of Oddi dysfunction will improve after endoscopic sphincterotomy, but some recommend that this subset of patients undergo cholescintigraphy or sphincter of Oddi manometry prior to sphincterotomy. Patients with type III biliary sphincter of Oddi dysfunction, who only have biliary pain, represent the most challenging subgroup. Medical and dietary treatment should be tried in conjunction with an extensive search for other causes, including functional bowel disease. If symptoms persist, cholescintigraphy or sphincter of Oddi manometry should be employed and endoscopic sphincterotomy performed sparingly after careful discussion. The majority of patients in this classification will not have abnormal findings on biliary manometry, and there is poor correlation between sphincter of Oddi manometry and response to sphincterotomy.

The responsiveness to endoscopic sphincterotomy for biliary sphincter of Oddi dysfunction varies based on subgroups of the Milwaukee classification. Most outcome studies report that up to 95% patients with type I sphincter of Oddi dysfunction are improved after sphincterotomy. About 60% of type II patients but only 15% of type III patients respond favorably. Most patients with type III sphincter of Oddi dysfunction show little improvement after sphincterotomy, because they do not meet any objective criteria for a definitive diagnosis of biliary sphincter of Oddi dysfunction. These patients should be evaluated extensively before performing any invasive diagnostic and therapeutic procedures unless they are experiencing severe and disabling biliary pain, structural abnormalities have been excluded, and they were unresponsive to trials of medical therapy.

Pancreatitis, the most frequent complication of endoscopic sphincterotomy, has a greater frequency when sphincterotomy is performed for functional biliary sphincter of Oddi disorders than for removal of common bile duct stones. This risk of pancreatitis increases more so in patients without common bile duct dilatation or with hypertensive pancreatic sphincter. Sphincter of Oddi dysfunction was an independent risk factor and tripled the risk of post-ERCP pancreatitis. Therefore, use of invasive diagnostic and therapeutic procedures in this functional condition are controversial, with some suggesting that the risk of complications exceeds the potential benefit. Endoscopic techniques are being developed to reduce the incidence of complications.

Functional Pancreatic Sphincter of Oddi Dysfunction

A number of reports now link motility disorders of the sphincter of Oddi to recurrent episodes of pancreatitis. Although randomized controlled trials are needed, total division of the sphincter of Oddi in patients with confirmed sphincter of Oddi dysfunction eliminates the episodes of recurrent pancreatitis. The majority of patients with recurrent episodes of acute pancreatitis due to pancreatic sphincter of Oddi dysfunction are female in their 40s which is a similar demographic for the incidence for biliary sphincter of Oddi dysfunction. Motility abnormalities of the pancreatic sphincter of Oddi are the most poorly understood of the functional disorders of the biliary tract and underlying physiologic evidence to explain the pathogenesis is lacking. Despite the potential for complications, manometry provides the most objective assessment of biliary sphincter of Oddi dysfunction, even though it only identifies only a small percentage of patients.

Clinical presentation: These patients present with intermittent episodes of epigastric pain that occur at intervals of up to months rather than days. Patients report that these episodes of pain, while not distinguishable from biliary-type pain, often radiate through to the back. The revised Rome guidelines propose that patients not only meet the criteria for

TABLE 17.6. Diagnostic criteria for functional pancreatic sphincter of Oddi disorder (Adapted from Behar J et al., 2006a. With permission by the Rome Foundation).

Must include both of the following:

1. Criteria for functional gallbladder and sphincter of Oddi disorder in Table 17.2

2. Elevated amylase/lipase

functional gallbladder and sphincter of Oddi disorder described in Table 17.2, but, in addition, that episodes of pain be associated with an increase in serum amylase and lipase and sometimes elevated liver enzymes or bilirubin depending on the severity of the pancreatitis (Table 17.6). Established etiologies of pancreatitis such as gallstones, alcohol abuse, pancreas divisum, or other causes of pancreatitis must be excluded before the diagnosis of a functional disorder should be considered. In addition to idiopathic recurrent pancreatitis, the differential diagnosis of microlithiasis and biliary sphincter of Oddi need to be considered.

Diagnostic evaluation: The algorithm for the diagnostic work-up of patients with biliary-type pain associated with increased pancreatic enzymes is shown in Fig. 17.4. Structural abnormalities such as microlithiasis or pancreas divisum must be excluded. The work-up, similar to that of biliary sphincter of Oddi disorder, is based on a comparable conservative tenet that non-invasive procedures be considered first. Depending on the patient's clinical presentation, the Rome guidelines propose that the most rational diagnostic sequence is that patients should undergo liver biochemistry and pancreatic enzymes followed by transabdominal ultrasonography, CT, EUS, and/or MRCP, and then, if necessary, diagnostic ERCP with bile analysis and sphincter of Oddi manometry as needed.

Although ultrasonography rarely shows any abnormalities during an episode of acute pancreatitis, it can be useful in monitoring the diameter of the pancreatic duct. Magnetic resonance cholangiopancreatography (MRCP) is becoming used more widely to evaluate the pancreatic duct in patients

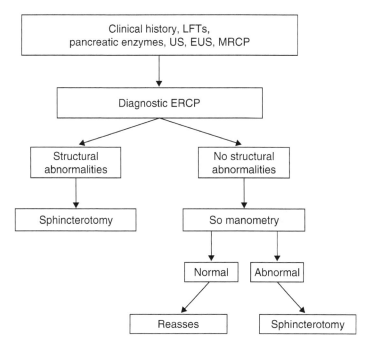

FIGURE 17.4. Algorithm of the diagnostic work-up and management of patients suspected with pancreatic sphincter of Oddi (SO) dysfunction. ERCP = endoscopic retrograde cholangiopancreatography (Reprinted from Behar J et al., 2006a. With permission by the Rome Foundation).

presenting with recurrent pancreatitis. Secretin infusion can be used to enhance the MR images of the pancreatic duct to detect abnormalities. EUS has also been used to explore for structural abnormalities and is perhaps most useful in identifying patients in whom a motility disorder of the sphincter may not be the primary cause of the pancreatitis. A classification similar to the Milwaukee types has been reported and includes pancreatic-type pain, amylase/lipase greater than 1.5–2 times normal, and pancreatic duct dilation greater than 5–6 mm (type I). Type II patients have pain and one of the other criteria, and type III patients only have pain. If ERCP finds no structural abnormalities, endoscopic manometry of both biliary and pancreatic sphincters is indicated (Fig. 17.4). Sphincter of Oddi manometry is perhaps the gold standard in selecting patients who will likely respond to the division of the sphincter. A manometric finding of excess sphincter of Oddi pressure does predict a successful outcome to surgical treatment. In patients with idiopathic recurrent pancreatitis, it is important to evaluate both the biliary and the pancreatic duct sphincters, because abnormalities in the pancreatic duct sphincter of Oddi may be detected in the presence of a normal biliary sphincter of Oddi manometry and vice versa. In some cases, the injection of Botox into the sphincter can be useful in selecting patients who will respond favorably to surgical division of the sphincter. The insertion of a stent into the pancreatic duct to facilitate drainage may also be used to select patients who may respond to sphincterotomy.

Treatment and outcome: Pharmacological agents have not been successful, and thus the best treatment for recurrent pancreatitis due to pancreatic sphincter of Oddi dysfunction is total surgical division of the sphincter of Oddi. Stenting of the pancreatic duct tends to be temporary and has not shown long-term benefits; however, it may be useful in identifying patients who will benefit from sphincterotomy. The complete surgical division ensures that both the biliary and the pancreatic sphincters are separated to allow free drainage of pancreatic juice and bile into the duodenum.

Surgical Approaches

Until the advent of endoscopic techniques, an open surgical approach was used to totally divide the sphincter of Oddi and the transampullary septum. Transduodenal sphincteroplasty and transampullary septectomy were the procedure of choice (Fig. 17.5a). Briefly, after a Kocher maneuver, a duodenotomy is made over the cannulated ampulla of Vater. After a sphincteroplasty, the transampullary septum is excised (Fig. 17.5b). Although restenosis occurs in up to 5% of patients, long-term

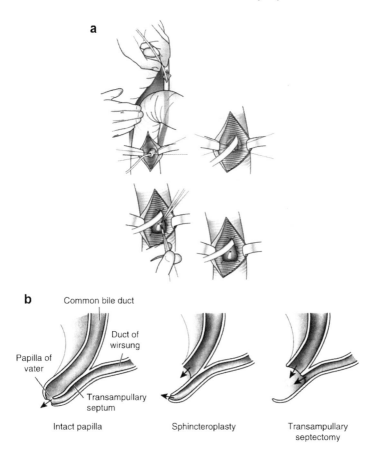

FIGURE 17.5. Abdominal approach to a Transduodenal Sphinc-teroplasty. (**a**) Steps in performing a transampullary septectomy in conjunction with a transduodenal sphincteroplasty. (**b**) Anatomic relationship within the papilla of Vater showing position of the amp-ullary septum forming the posterior wall of the bile duct and the anterior wall of the duct of Wirsung (Reprinted from Desai et al., 2004. Copyright 2004. With permission from Elsevier).

follow-up suggests reasonable resolution of symptoms. Should restenosis occur, a stent can be inserted endoscopically to reestablish flow. More recently, endoscopic techniques have

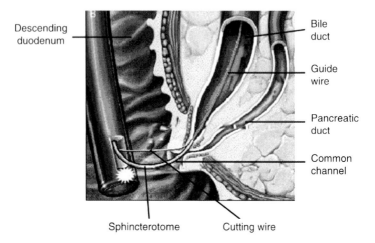

Descending duodenum

Bile duct

Guide wire

Pancreatic duct

Common channel

Sphincterotome   Cutting wire

FIGURE 17.6. Endoscopic sphincterotomy. A standard sphinctero-tomy requires successful retrograde cannulation of the bile duct (shown in example) or pancreatic duct. Once access is confirmed radiographically, a guide wire is passed into the duct and the sphincter is incised by means of electrocautery through a traction-type papil-lotome, with the cutting wire bowed against the roof of the papilla (Reprinted from Freeman et al., 1996. Copyright 1996 Massachusetts Medical Society. With permission. All rights reserved).

been developed to divide both biliary and pancreatic duct sphincters. The procedure entails the selective cannulation of bile and pancreatic ducts followed by the division of the sphincter by use of a sphincterotomy (Fig. 17.6). Although the efficacy of the endoscopic procedure is comparable to the open approach, no long-term results will validate the superiority of either approach; thus, endoscopic sphincterotomy has become the technique of choice. Complications of endoscopic sphinc-terotomy include pancreatitis, bleeding, perforation, and infec-tion which can range in severity from mild to life-threatening. Paying close attention to technique and taking measures to minimize risk, recognition, and immediate management of complications will reduce the incidence but not eliminate all adverse outcomes. As with any invasive procedure, complication rates are substantially lower when the procedure is performed by an experienced surgeon or endoscopist with a high volume of procedures.

Even though there are purported benefits to the patient, endoscopic pancreatic sphincterotomy is practiced less widely than endoscopic biliary sphincterotomy. Despite a higher complication rate, pancreatic sphincterotomy is safe and effective when used as primary therapy, although pancreatic drainage has been suggested to reduce the incidence of pancreatitis. Overnight nasopancreatic drainage is the method of choice, because it carries a complication rate as low as stent placement, but without the need for a repeat procedure, and presumably without the risk of ductal and parenchymal damage.

Selected Readings

Barnes SL, Clark DM, Schwartz RW, (2004) Biliary dyskinesia: a brief review. Curr Surg 61:428–434

Behar J, Corazziari E, Guelrud M, et al. (2006a) Functional gallbladder and sphincter of Oddi disorders In: Drossman DA et al. (eds) Rome III: functional gastrointestinal disorders, 3rd edn. Degnon, McLean, VA, pp 595–638

Behar J et al. (2006b) Functional gallbladder and sphincter of Oddi disorders. Gastroenterology 130:1498–1509

Boyden EA, (1957) The anatomy of the choledochoduodenal junction in man. Surg Gynecol Obstet 104:641

Desai KM, et al. (2004) Postcholecystectomy problems. In: Cameron JL (ed) Current surgical therapy, 8th edn

Freeman ML, Guda NM (2005) Endoscopic biliary and pancreatic sphincterotomy. Curr Treat Options Gastroenterol 8:127–134

Freeman ML, et al. (1996) Complications of endoscopic sphincterotomy. N Engl J Med 335:909–918

Funch-Jensen P, Drewes AM, Madacsy L (2006) Evaluation of the biliary tract in patients with functional biliary symptoms. World J Gastroenterol 12:2839–2845

Moody FG, Berenson MM, McCloskey D (1977) Transampullary septectomy for post-cholecystectomy pain. Ann Surg 186:415–423

Prajapati DN, Hogan WJ (2003) Sphincter of Oddi dysfunction and other functional biliary disorders: evaluation and treatment. Gastroenterol Clin North Am 32:601–618

Rosenblatt ML, Catalano MF, Alcocer E, Geenen JE (2001) Comparison of sphincter of Oddi manometry, fatty meal sonography, and hepatobiliary scintigraphy in the diagnosis of sphincter of Oddi dysfunction. Gastrointest Endosc 54:697–704

Sgouros SN, Pereira SP (2006) Systematic review: sphincter of Oddi dysfunction – non-invasive diagnostic methods and long-term outcome after endoscopic sphincterotomy. Aliment Pharmacol Ther 24:237–246

Tarnasky PR, Palesch YY, Cunningham JT, et al. (1998) Pancreatic stenting prevents pancreatitis after biliary sphincterotomy in patients with sphincter of Oddi dysfunction. Gastroenterology 115:1518–1524

Toouli J (2002) Biliary dyskinesia. Curr Treat Options Gastroenterol 5:285–291

18
Primary Sclerosing Cholangitis

Nicholas J. Zyromski and Henry A. Pitt

Pearls and Pitfalls

- With sclerosing cholangitis, strictures involve the extrahepatic bile ducts exclusively in 10% of patients, solely the intrahepatic bile ducts in 15%, and both intrahepatic and extrahepatic bile ducts in 75%.
- Cholangiocarcinoma (CCA) develops in 8–18% of patients with primary sclerosing cholangitis (PSC); the diagnosis of CCA is made concurrently with that of PSC in 40–60% of patients.
- The diagnosis of CCA in the presence of PSC is notoriously difficult; biliary brushings and cytology have a sensitivity of less than 40%.
- Repeated endoscopic therapy of dominant strictures may delay the diagnosis of CCA and affect survival adversely.
- Operative resection of dominant extrahepatic strictures may prevent development of CCA, prolong survival, and delay need for liver transplantation.
- Once cirrhosis develops, liver transplantation is the optimal therapy for patients with PSC; outcomes are equivalent to, or better than, those of transplantation for other indications.
- Approximately 70% of patients with PSC also have inflammatory bowel disease (IBD); therefore, screening colonoscopy should be employed routinely (even for patients who do not carry the diagnosis of IBD).

K.I. Bland et al. (eds.), *Liver and Biliary Surgery*,
DOI 10.1007/978-1-84996-429-6_18,
© Springer-Verlag London Limited 2011

Introduction

PSC is an uncommon but important disease that manifests as inflammatory strictures affecting both the intrahepatic and extrahepatic biliary tree to varying degrees. About 75% of patients with PSC have stricturing of both intrahepatic and extrahepatic bile ducts, with 15% having only intrahepatic and 10% having only extrahepatic involvement of the bile duct. The prevalence of PSC in Western countries is approximately 8 per 100,000. The pathophysiology of PSC is poorly understood, and the clinical course of the disease is widely variable. The disease, however, is monotonously progressive, leading to cholestasis, hepatic cirrhosis, and death from liver failure if hepatic transplantation is not performed. The median survival from time of diagnosis to liver transplantation or death is 12–18 years.

Approximately 70% of patients with PSC also have IBD, and 10–20% of PSC patients will develop CCA – an important consideration when formulating treatment plans. No medical therapy delays progression of the disease or prolongs overall or transplant-free survival. Once hepatic cirrhosis has developed, liver transplantation is the treatment of choice. A wide variety of percutaneous, endoscopic, and operative therapies have been applied to patients with dominant biliary strictures; however, no level I data are available to compare these options properly. In select patients with dominant extrahepatic strictures, complete operative resection may prevent development of CCA, prolong survival, and delay the need for liver transplantation.

Associated Diseases

Approximately 70% of patients with PSC also have IBD, predominantly ulcerative colitis. Only 10% of all patients with IBD, however, develop PSC. About 75% of patients will be diagnosed with IBD before the diagnosis of PSC is established. In some patients, however, the diagnosis of IBD manifests only after liver transplantation for PSC. All patients with the diagnosis of PSC should therefore undergo routine

TABLE 18.1. Associated diseases in primary sclerosing cholangitis.

Inflammatory bowel disease

Cholangiocarcinoma

Ankylosing spondylitis

Autoimmune thyroiditis

Celiac disease

Pancreatitis

Colon adenocarcinoma

Pancreatic adenocarcinoma

colonoscopy (even in the absence of a diagnosis of IBD). A number of other autoimmune diseaseshave been associated, albeit less commonly, with PSC, including ankylosing spondylitis, autoimmune thyroiditis, andceliac disease. Patients with PSC are also at a moderately increased risk for developing pancreatitis, pancreatic adenocarcinoma, and colorectal adenocarcinoma (Table 18.1).

CCA develops in 8–18% of patients with PSC and is the second leading cause of death after liver failure in most series. This increased incidence – greater than 150 times that in the general population – coupled with the generally poor outcome and notorious difficulty in diagnosis (see below) makes CCA the most feared complication of PSC. About half of patients with CCA are diagnosed either concurrently or within 1 year of the diagnosis of PSC. CCA occurs more frequently in women and in the setting of IBD; however, no clear correlation exists between the duration of PSC or development of hepatic cirrhosis and the development of CCA.

Pathophysiology

The precise pathophysiology of PSC is poorly understood but remains an area of active basic and clinical research. Laboratory investigation has been hampered by the lack of an animal model that reproduces accurately the course and outcome of the disease. A genetic component is likely, as siblings of PSC patients have a 100-fold predisposition to develop PSC. The inheritance pattern is complex, and no common mutation has yet been identified. The idea that PSC is an autoimmune disease is enticing, because multiple autoantibodies such as antinuclear antibody (ANA) have been associated with PSC. While a dysregulation of the immune system appears to play a role in the development of PSC, no direct evidence documents that PSC is an auto-immune disease. Current research is focused on the basic biology of the cholangiocyte, including epithelial transporter proteins and the response to an inflammatory insult. Other promising basic research uses gene knockout technology in attempts to create a functional animal model of PSC.

Clinical Presentation

PSC most commonly affects Caucasian males with an aver-age age at diagnosis of 42 years. The clinical presentation is widely variable. Many patients present with jaundice and/or pruritus, and at least half will report right upper quadrant pain and fatigue at the time of diagnosis. In some instances, PSC will be diagnosed by the finding of increased serum liver chemistry tests on routine screening of patients with IBD. True cholangitis (i.e., infection with fever and chills) is very rare prior to manipulation of the biliary tree. Some of the 15% of patients with isolated small duct disease will present with typical signs and symptoms of end-stage liver disease.

Diagnosis

Endoscopic retrograde cholangiography (ERC) remains the gold standard for diagnosing PSC. In experienced hands, ERC demonstrates accurately the intrahepatic and extrahepatic biliary tree more than 95% of the time. This direct imaging modality also offers the potential to provide therapy by balloon dilatation and/or stenting of dominant strictures, as well as the ability to obtain bile and cytologic brushings (though the accuracy of cytology for diagnosing CCA is poor). The obvious disadvantage of ERC is its invasiveness, with a small but real potential for complications, including cholangitis, bleeding, perforation of the biliary tree, and pancreatitis. Additionally, visualization of the intrahepatic biliary tree proximal to high-grade strictures may be technically difficult.

Magnetic resonance cholangiography (MRC) is a noninvasive alternative to ERC for the diagnosis of PSC (Fig. 18.1). Magnetic resonance technology has improved dramatically over the past decade, and many high-volume centers currently

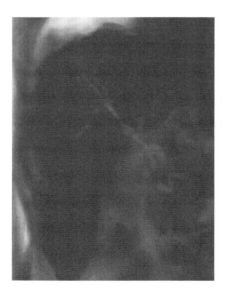

FIGURE 18.1. Magnetic resonance cholangiogram in a patient with primary sclerosing cholangitis demonstrating multiple intrahepatic strictures with a dominant extrahepatic stricture. Note cirrhotic liver and presence of ascites above liver.

use this noninvasive imaging modality routinely for screening and follow-up of patients with PSC because it allows accurate imaging of the entire biliary tree, including intrahepatic ducts proximal to strictures and provides cross-sectional images of the liver, its vasculature, and the rest of the abdomen. MRC is purely a diagnostic test.

Percutaneous transhepatic cholangiography (PTC) provides, albeit invasively, direct ductal visualization of the biliary tree via a proximal approach and, similar to ERC, affords the potential for therapy by dilatation and/or stenting of dominant strictures. The stents placed at the time of PTC are by necessity internal/external. In the setting of PSC with multiple intrahepatic strictures, PTC is a challenging procedure even for the most experienced interventional radiologist; currently, PTC is reserved for highly selected patients.

The specter of CCA looms large in the setting of PSC; unfortunately, the diagnosis of biliary malignancy in the face of multiple strictures is notoriously difficult. Despite rigorous preoperative screening, incidental CCA is found in 3–9% of livers explanted from patients undergoing hepatic transplantation for PSC, highlighting this difficulty. Clinical symptoms of increasing abdominal pain, jaundice, and weight loss are nonspecific and mimic many of the symptoms related to progression of benign strictures.

The gold standard for making the diagnosis of CCA in the setting of PSC is tissue histology. Unfortunately, the accuracy of biliary brushings and biopsy obtained at the time of ERC is less than 40%. False-positive results may occur with indwelling stents, and a negative cytologic diagnosis does not exclude the diagnosis of CCA.

Cross-sectional abdominal imaging by computed tomography (CT) or magnetic resonance imaging (MRI) is mandatory in the follow-up of patients with PSC; however, the accuracy of these tests in detecting CCA is poor. The role of positron emission tomography (PET) for the diagnosis of CCA in PSC is evolving, but the early studies have shown poor sensitivity and specificity.

Serum markers, such as carbohydrate antigen (CA) 19-9 and carcinogenic embryonic antigen (CEA), also have been evaluated. While CA 19-9 is relatively specific for diagnosing CCA, this test lacks sensitivity and may be spuriously elevated in the jaundiced patient.

Approximately 80% of biliary malignancies are associated with chromosomal abnormalities. Digital image analysis (DIA) and fluorescence in situ hybridization (FISH) are sophisticated cytologic techniques that diagnose malignancy by identifying chromosomal abnormalities (Fig. 18.2). Both DIA and FISH technology have been applied recently to the diagnosis of CCA in PSC. Preliminary studies in small numbers

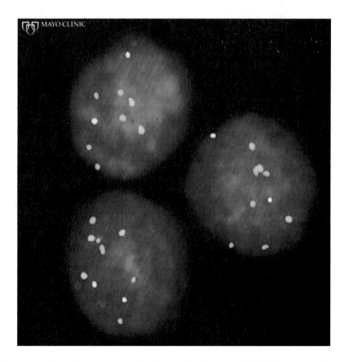

FIGURE 18.2. Fluorescence in situ hybridization (FISH) demonstrating multiple polysomies in a patient with cholangiocarcinoma (Courtesy of Michael J. Levy, MD, Mayo Clinic).

of patients have shown promise but require validation with larger groups.

Therefore, a high index of suspicion is paramount to secure the diagnosis of CCA. Complete operative resection offers the best chance of survival for these patients. Patients with recurrent dominant strictures and those with cellular atypia or dysplasia on biopsy or brushing are best evaluated with operative exploration rather than repeated attempts at endoscopic diagnosis.

Medical Therapy

Numerous medical therapies have been tried in patients with PSC, including antifibrotic agents, immunosuppressants such as corticosteroids, tacrolimus (FK 506), and Methotrexate, mitotic inhibitors (Colchicine), antibiotics, and inhibitors of tumor necrosis factor alpha (TNF-α). To date, unfortunately, no medical therapy has been shown to delay progression of disease, prolong survival or time until need for liver transplantation, or improve overall outcomes in patients with PSC. The hydrophilic bile acid ursodexoycholic acid (UDCA) and glucocorticosteroids are two of the most widely studied agents. Prospective, randomized trials of UDCA administration to patients with PSC have demonstrated improvements in liver chemistry values but have failed to improve liver histology, need for transplantation, or overall survival. Similarly, prospective trials of corticosteroids have failed to demonstrate objective improvement in the outcome of patients with PSC. In addition, glucocorticoids should be used cautiously, because they may mask symptoms of biliary infection and may actually increase the infectious risk. Several clinical trials are underway currently focusing on targeted therapy.

Liver Transplantation

Once hepatic cirrhosis has developed in the setting of PSC, liver transplantation is the optimal therapy. Approximately 5% of all liver transplants in the USA are performed for end-stage liver disease secondary to PSC. The technical conduct of liver transplantation for PSC is similar to that for other causes of end-stage liver disease, with the exception that the extrahepatic biliary tree is resected in its entirety down to the head of the pancreas, and the donor bile duct is reconstructed with a Roux-en-Y limb of the recipient jejunum. Previous biliary surgery has not been shown to affect the outcome of liver transplantation for PSC.

As noted above, despite rigorous preoperative screening, unsuspected CCA is found in 3–9% of the explanted livers with PSC. Interesting data from two large series of liver transplantation have suggested that if these "incidental" CCA are less than 1 cm in size, long-term survival is not decreased. In these same series, however, patients with known CCA at the time of liver transplantation had dramatically worse outcomes. It should be highlighted, therefore, that outside of established investigational protocols with aggressive screening and preoperative chemoradiation, the known presence of CCA remains a contraindication to liver transplantation.

The optimal timing of liver transplantation in PSC remains an unresolved question. Outcomes are improved if liver transplantation is performed prior to the development of cirrhosis. The overall goals of early transplantation are to reduce the risk of CCA, improve survival, and reduce the overall cost of therapy. As most CCAs are diagnosed within 1 year of the diagnosis of PSC, early transplantation would play only a small (4%) role in prevention and would not improve overall survival over 5 years. Additionally, early transplantation would increase the costs of medical care by 2–3 times. Therefore, a treatment algorithm that includes early transplantation for the 10% of patients with established cirrhosis, biliary surgery for patients with dominant extrahepatic strictures (10%), or suspicion of CCA (10%) and late transplantation for low and moderate-risk patients (70%) appears to be warranted.

Aggressive protocols of colonoscopic screening are indicated for PSC patients after liver transplantation, because up to 15% of patients with IBD will develop colon cancer within 5 years after liver transplantation. Although UDCA is administered commonly to IBD patients after transplant in efforts to prevent development of colon cancer, little objective evidence supports this practice.

Therapy of Dominant Strictures

Non-operative management. Both endoscopic and percutaneous transhepatic approaches have been used to treat dominant biliary strictures. Recently, most tertiary centers have favored the endoscopic approach. Up to 80% of patients demonstrate a clinical response to endoscopic therapy of dominant strictures. Prospective studies of endoscopic balloon dilatation alone versus dilatation and stenting have failed to demonstrate benefit from stenting. The rates of stent occlusion and cholangitis are high, and routine stent placement in the setting of PSC has fallen out of favor. The major complications of endoscopic therapy include bleeding, perforation, cholangitis, and pancreatitis, almost all of which are amenable to medical management. No prospective series has yet compared endoscopic to operative therapy in the treatment of dominant strictures. A persistent concern with prolonged endoscopic therapy is the delay in diagnosis of CCA.

Operative resection. In the absence of cirrhosis, resection of dominant extrahepatic strictures provides durable relief of jaundice, confirms or excludes the diagnosis of CCA, and delays the progression of hepatic cirrhosis and need for liver transplantation. Preoperative evaluation includes high-quality abdominal CT with both arterial and venous phase images. This workup allows accurate evaluation of hepatic vascular anatomy, including common variations, as well as assessment of liver atrophy/hypertrophy. Percutaneous transhepatic stents are placed routinely in both right and left hepatic ducts, facilitating markedly the intraoperative dissection of the hepatic bifurcation. Perioperative antibiotics are tailored to cover specific bacteria cultured from the bile. Figure 18.3 depicts the general operative approach to resection of the extrahepatic biliary tree. An upper midline incision provides

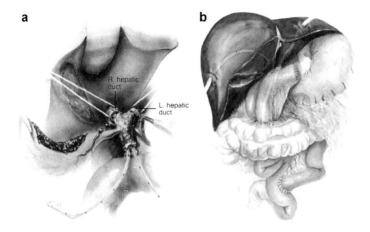

FIGURE 18.3. Operative approach to resection of the extrahepatic biliary tree (Reprinted from Cameron, 1990. With permission).

excellent exposure, and facilitates optimal placement of transhepatic stents on the abdominal wall. Thorough abdominal exploration includes routine intraoperative ultrasonography of the liver and porta hepatis. Suspicious liver nodules and lymph nodes are biopsied for frozen section analysis. Despite complete preoperative workup, including tumor markers, cytology, and adequate imaging, unsuspected malignant disease is encountered occasionally. Therefore, the surgeon should be prepared to undertake an extended resection (including hepatectomy) should a malignancy be found.

After abdominal exploration, the hepatic flexure of the colon is mobilized off the head of the pancreas and a generous Kocher maneuver performed. After cholecystectomy, the common bile duct is divided close to the head of the pancreas, and the distal common bile duct is over sewn. At this point, a frozen section of the distal margin should be reviewed by an experienced pathologist. The proximal bile duct is dissected from the porta hepatis, taking care to preserve the right hepatic artery, which generally dives posterior to the common hepatic duct. The right and left hepatic ducts are divided proximal to the dominant stricture, and intraoperative frozen section analysis of the proximal margin is performed to exclude malignancy. The preoperatively placed transhepatic stents are then exchanged retrograde for large, soft Silastic catheters. A Roux limb of jejunum is brought through the mesocolon to the right of the middle colic vessels, and the anastomoses are created over the Silastic catheters. Chromic sutures are placed in the liver around the exit sites of the stents to minimize bile leakage and venous ooze. The Silastic stents are passed through the abdominal wall away from the midline incision, incorporating a gentle curve to avoid kinking and to aid postoperative stent exchange. Intraoperative cholangiography confirms proper stent position and excludes anastomotic leak. This maneuver is facilitated by placement of an atraumatic bowel clamp on the Roux limb distal to the stents. After cholangiography, contrast is aspirated to minimize intrabiliary pressure and bacterial translocation.

Postoperative management is similar to that for any major abdominal procedure. Intraoperative stent manipulation and cholangiography creates mild cholangitis; thus, antibiotics are continued postoperatively until the patient remains afebrile for 24 h. Transhepatic stents are exchanged under radiologic guidance at 3-month intervals. The duration of postoperative stenting is individualized on the basis of specific anatomy and postoperative clinical course. In most patients, these stents can be removed. When removal is contemplated, the Whittaker test is performed to document intrabiliary pressure, and a good quality cholangiogram is performed. In the absence of increased biliary pressure or anastomotic stricture, the stents may are removed.

Outcomes

Liver transplantation. Long-term survival after liver transplantation for PSC is excellent. Several series have documented 5-year patient survival of 80–85% and 5-year graft survival of 70–75%. These overall outcomes are somewhat better than those of liver transplantation performed for other indications; however, patients undergoing liver transplantation for PSC have a modestly higher complication rate. Hepatic artery thrombosis is more common in the setting of PSC and often requires re-transplantation. Patients undergoing liver transplantation for PSC have a higher re-transplant rate at 2 years (10%) versus those patients transplanted for other indications (5%). Acute cellular rejection, chronic ductopenic rejection, and biliary strictures all occur with more frequency in patients undergoing liver transplant for PSC.

Recurrent PSC in the transplanted liver is a vexing problem and may occur in as many as one third of patients. The true incidence of recurrent PSC is difficult to define accurately due to wide variability in diagnostic criteria and follow-up. Similarly, whether recurrence of PSC in the transplanted liver affects long-term outcome directly is unclear.

Endoscopic therapy. A recent report from Indiana University is representative of outcomes of endoscopic therapy of dominant strictures in PSC. In this large series, 63 patients were treated endoscopically over a 6-year time period with a median follow-up of 34 months. Sixty-one patients underwent balloon dilatation a mean of 2.3 times, and 53% had a temporary biliary stent placed. Seven patients died (5 from liver failure, 2 from CCA) and eight underwent liver transplantation. CCA was diagnosed in five patients (8%) in this series. The overall 1-, 3-, and 5-year survival (97%, 87%, and 83%) was greater (p <0.05) than predicted (92%, 77%, and 65%). The authors concluded appropriately that these results should be viewed with caution, because they provide only indirect evidence that endoscopic stenting improves survival in patients with PSC and dominant strictures.

Operative resection. A large series from Johns Hopkins evaluated the outcomes of 146 patients with PSC managed by resection, percutaneous or endoscopic balloon dilatation, medical therapy alone, or liver transplantation. In the absence of cirrhosis, overall 5-year survival and transplant-free survival was greater (p <0.05) in patients undergoing resection versus those managed endoscopically or percutaneously (overall survival 85% versus 59%, transplant-free survival 82% versus 46%) (Fig. 18.4). Patients with cirrhosis had longer survival after liver transplantation than after resection or

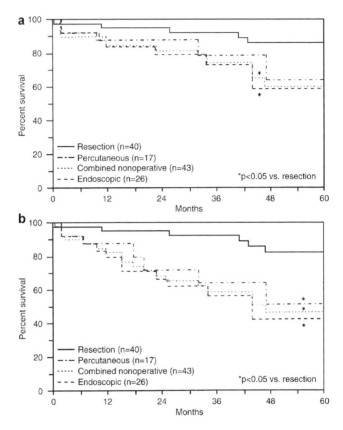

FIGURE 18.4. Overall **(a)** and transplant-free **(b)** survival in non-cirrhotic patients with PSC undergoing resection, endoscopic, or percutaneous therapy (Reprinted from Ahrendt et al., 1998. With permission of Lippincott Williams & Wilkins).

endoscopic management. Importantly, CCA developed in 6% of the endoscopic/percutaneous group and in none of the patients managed by resection.

Overall morbidity after operative resection of the extrahepatic biliary tree is 30–40%, and perioperative mortality is about 3%. Complications specific to the biliary tree include cholangitis, hemobilia, and bile leak, almost all of which are amenable to nonoperative management.

Summary

PSC is a poorly understood, progressive disease causing strictures of the biliary tree and resulting in cholestasis, hepatic cirrhosis, and death from liver failure. Approximately 70% of patients with PSC also have IBD. No medical therapy will alter the course of the disease. Endoscopic cholangiography remains the gold standard for diagnosis, though MRC techniques have improved, and this test is used routinely for surveillance. The clinician must maintain a high degree of suspicion for CCA, which develops in 10–20% of patients with PSC. Malignant biliary strictures are notoriously difficult to diagnose. Endoscopic therapy with balloon dilatation of dominant strictures is employed in many patients, but patients with recurrent dominant strictures or a suspicion for CCA should undergo operative exploration. In selected patients without cirrhosis, resection of the extrahepatic biliary tree confirms or excludes CCA and provides durable therapy. In the setting of cirrhosis, liver transplantation is the optimal therapy. Current research is directed toward better understanding the biology of PSC, identifying medical therapy, and developing more sensitive diagnostic techniques for CCA.

Selected Readings

Ahrendt SA, Pitt HA, Kalloo AN, et al. (1998) Primary sclerosing cholangitis: resect, dilate, or transplant? Ann Surg 227:412–423

Ahrendt SA, Pitt HA, Nakeeb A, et al. (1999) Diagnosis and management of cholangiocarcinoma in primary sclerosing cholangitis. J Gastrointest Surg 3:357–368

Baluyut AR, Sherman S, Lehman GA, et al. (2001) Impact of endoscopic therapy on the survival of patients with primary sclerosing cholangitis. Gastrointest Endosc 53:308–312

Cameron J (1990) Atlas of surgery, vol. 1. BC Decker, Philadelphia

Cameron JL, Pitt HA, Zinner MJ, et al. (1988) Resection of hepatic duct bifurcation and transhepatic stenting for sclerosing cholangitis. Ann Surg 207:614–622

Graziadei IW, Weisner RH, Marotta PJ, et al. (1999) Long-term results of patients undergoing liver transplantation for primary sclerosing cholangitis. Hepatology 30:1121–1127

Part IV
Biliary—Malignant

19

Perihilar Cholangiocarcinoma

Yuji Nimura and Hideki Nishio

Pearls and Pitfalls

- Surgical resection remains the only opportunity for survival and is mandatory.
- Do not abandon surgical resection prior to establishing definite contraindication, even when resection is technically difficult.
- Surgical resection is possible in approximately 70% of patients with Bismuth type IV tumor.
- Confirm accurate surgical anatomy to precisely, assess surgical indications allowing for complete surgical resection.
- Surgical resection of hilar cholangiocarcinoma is required to obviate complicated biliary obstructions.
- Segmental hepatectomy combined with caudate lobectomy, extrahepatic bile duct resection and extended lymphadenectomy are standard components of the surgical procedure.
- Aggressive surgery inclusive of portal vein resection and reconstruction for invasion of the portal vein offers survival superior to that of conservative therapy.
- Liver functions must be carefully evaluated *prior* to surgery as obstructive jaundice impairs hepatic function.
- Perioperative management is essential to perform safe, extended hepatectomy for biliary cancer patients.

K.I. Bland et al. (eds.), *Liver and Biliary Surgery*,
DOI 10.1007/978-1-84996-429-6_19,
© Springer-Verlag London Limited 2011

Introduction

Perihilar cholangiocarcinoma includes extrahepatic and intrahepatic cholangiocarcinomas that involve the hepatic confluence of the bile duct. Although this intractable disease used to bedifficult to resect as a result of complex anatomy of the hepatic hilum, diagnostic and surgical strategy has changed drastically over the past two decades. Hepatobiliary resection based on precise preoperative diagnosis of tumor extent has become a standard procedure to obtain curative resection. Despite the advance of preoperative diagnostic techniques, perihilar cholangiocarcinomais typically diagnosed in an advanced stage at initial presentation. As only surgical resection can offer the superior survival probability, combined portal vein and liver resection and/or hepatopancreatoduodenectomy are aggressively performed at leading centers. In this chapter, we describe the clinical outline of perihilar cholangiocarcinoma and our recommendation for treating this intractable tumor.

Clinical Presentation

Most patients appear with obstructive jaundice. Even in patients without jaundice, serum alkaline phosphatase and/or γ-glutamyltranspeptidase are usually elevated. Those symptoms result from bile congestion due to biliary stricture of the hepatic confluence involved by advanced cholangiocarcinoma. Ultrasonography is performed in those patients and reveals dilated intrahepatic bile ducts, the normal or atrophic gallbladder and sometimes a tumor itself, suggesting perihilar cholangiocarcinoma. Computed tomography (CT) or magnetic resonance imaging (MRI) is carried out for further examination. As CT or MRI usually indicate which lobe of the liver is predominantly involved, biliary drainage is applied to decompress the future remnant hepatic lobe.

Diagnosis

Advanced perihilar cholangiocarcinoma thickens the bile duct wall, resulting in biliary stricture. Therefore, the extent of biliary stricture is evaluated carefully to diagnose tumor extent along the bile duct. For this purpose, direct cholangiography via the biliary drainage catheters remains the best modality and provides advanced resolution of the images. As intrahepatic bile ducts run three dimensionally, they superimpose upon each other in two-dimensional cholangiograms. Therefore, direct cholangiography should be utilized in several projections to avoid superimposition of the intrahepatic bile ducts. Confluence patterns of the intrahepatic segmental ducts, which differs in each patient, should be evaluated in detail as well as tumor extent along the bile duct. After consideration of this information, resection planes of the intrahepatic bile ducts is planned (Fig. 19.1). As the *type of hepatectomy* determines the resection

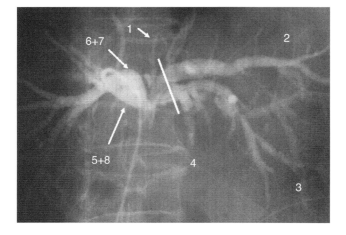

FIGURE 19.1. Right anterior oblique view of direct cholangiography through a PTBD catheter. Stenosis of the hepatic confluence is demonstrated. Resection line of the intrahepatic bile ducts is planed as shown by a white solid line. 1, caudate lobe branch of the bile duct; 2, left lateral posterior segmental bile duct; 3, left lateral anterior segmental bile duct; 4, left medial sectional bile duct; 5 + 8, right anterior sectional bile duct; 6 + 7 right posterior sectional bile duct.

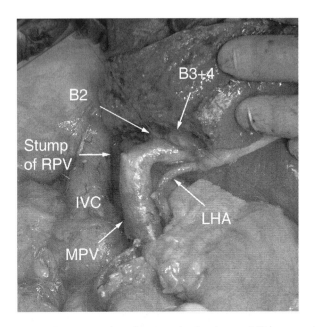

FIGURE 19.2. Intraoperative photograph after hepatobiliary resection (same patient as in Fig. 19.1). Stumps of the left lateral posterior segmental bile duct (B2) and the trunk of the left lateral anterior segmental and the left medial sectional bile duct (B3 + 4) are shown on the liver transection plane. The transection plane is consistent with the resection line of the intrahepatic bile ducts which was planed preoperatively. RPV, right portal vein; IVC, inferior vena cava; LHA, left hepatic artery; MPV, main portal vein.

line for the intrahepatic bile ducts, following planning of this plane, the type of hepatectomy is automatically determined in most patients. As it is impossible to diagnose tumor extent intraoperatively, preoperative precise diagnosis of tumor extent is critically important in the evaluation process. The consistency between a resection line of the bile ducts and the preoperative plan is intraoperatively confirmed (Figs. 19.1 and 19.2).

Cancer infiltration in the hepatoduodenal ligament is estimated by multidetector row-computed tomography (MDCT, Figs. 19.3 and 19.4). Previously, we performed hepatic

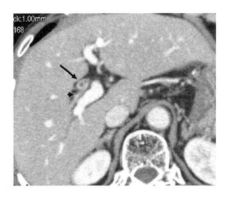

FIGURE 19.3. Axial view of multiplanar reformation image of pos-tenhanced multidetector row computed tomography. Thickened wall of the proximal bile duct is enhanced (arrow) and adherent to the right hepatic artery (arrow head).

arteriography and percutaneous transhepatic portography to evaluate distribution and cancer invasion of the vessels in the hepatoduodenal ligament. However, the recent advance of MDCT offers finely reconstructed images: multiplanar refor-mation (MPR); volume rendered (VR); and maximum inten-sity projection (MIP) images, to obtain adequate information in a non-invasive way (Figs. 19.3 and 19.4). Combination portal vein and liver resection for locally advanced cancer that invades the portal vein is performed at leading centers. Therefore, when MPR images demonstrate portal vein inva-sion, we evaluate the location and extent of the portal vein invasion and predicate the design of resection (segmental or wedge) and reconstruction (direct anastomosis or autogenous vein grafting) procedures with guidance based on findings on VR or MIP images. Perineural invasion, lymph node metastasis and liver metastasis are also estimated by MPR images. Coronal view of MPR image is quite useful for this purpose.

As perihilar cholangiocarcicoma often requires major resection of a cholestatic liver to obtain curative resection, septic morbidity followed by liver failure is one of the seri-ous postoperative complications and may result in a fatal condition. Therefore, preoperative liver function must be

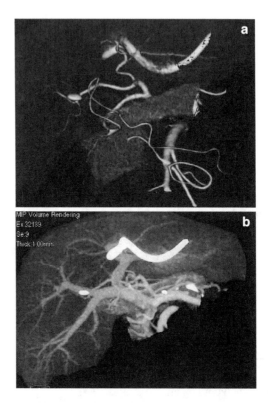

FIGURE 19.4. Three dimensional images to evaluate distribution and extent of cancer invasion of the vessels in the hepatoduodenal ligament. (**a**) Caudal oblique view of volume rendered image. (**b**) Caudal oblique view of maximum intensity projection image.

estimated carefully. We examine indocyanine green (ICG) test, calculate the liver volume using CT, and determine plasma disappearance rate of ICG multiplying % volume of the future remnant liver >0.05 to be a surgical indication.

Perioperative Management

After surgical resection of perihilar cholangiocarcinoma, septic complications followed by liver failure may cause hospital death. Therefore, perioperative management to avoid such fatal complications is most important. Although the necessity of biliary drainage for obstructive jaundice before hepatectomy is still controversial, percutaneous transhepatic (PTBD) or endoscopic nasal biliary drainage (ENBD) is completed in most patients who are to undergo hepatobiliary resection. As perihilar cholangiocarcinoma causes complex biliary stricture, additional PTBD is often required even in patients who had already undergone ENBD because of insufficient drainage or obstructive segmental cholangitis. Endoscopic retrograde biliary drainage should not be completed due to the high incidence of cholangitis; its value is greatly limited in diagnosing tumor extent along the bile duct. Metallic stent should not be placed in patients with potentially resectable tumor. Major hepatectomy is performed after total serum bilirubin decreases to <2 mg/dl.

Percutaneous transhepatic portal embolization (PTPE) should be carried out to enlarge the future remnant liver in patients who will undergo right or more extensive hepatectomy. As bile replacement during external biliary drainage can restore the intestinal barrier function in patients with biliary obstruction and may reduce bacterial translocation, externally drained bile should be replaced orally or through a nasoduodenal tube before surgery and through a feeding catheter placed intraoperatively after surgery. Synbiotics should also be given as they can reduce postoperative infectious complications.

Treatment

As only surgical resection can offer a chance of long-term survival in patients with perihilar cholangiocarcoinoma, aggressive surgery is recommended even for locally advanced perihilar cholangiocarcinoma. As R0 resection can rarely be obtained for bile duct resection without hepatectomy, segmental hepatectomy combined with caudate lobe resection, extrahepatic bile duct resection, and extended lymphadenectomy is the standard procedure. Type of hepatectomy should be determined according to cancer extent along the bile duct diagnosed by direct cholangiography (Fig. 19.1). Surgical

indication should not be determined based on Bismuth classification alone as surgical resection could be carried out in
approximately 70% of patients with Bismuth type IV tumor
in the authors' unit. Portal vein invasion is not a surgical contraindication at leading centers. Right hepatic artery invasion
also is not a contraindication for surgical resection in cases
of left-sided hepatectomy. Hepatopancreatoduodenectomy
(major hepatectomy and pancreatoduodenectomy) is indicated for a locally-advanced tumor invading both the hepatic
confluence and the intrapancreatic bile duct. The presence of
para-aortic lymph node metastasis may not be a surgical contraindication in selected patients. Although liver transplantation has been performed, its value remains controversial
when compared with surgical resection.

Outcome

Resection rate varies from 19% to 89% according to centers
in the world. In the authors', resection rate was 76% (351/461
patients, 1977–2005) and R0 resection was possible in 70%
among the resected patients (246/351 patients). Overall
5-year survival rate and median survival time were 22% and
2 years, respectively.

Our recent multivariate analyses revealed histologic differentiation (moderate/poor), positive lymph node metastasis
and macroscopic portal vein invasion are independent negative prognostic factors of survival. Five-year survival rates for
patients with and without lymph node metastasis, and for
patients with and without portal vein resection were 10% and
34%, and 11% and 27%, respectively. Five-year survival rate
and median survival time for patients with R0 resection were
27% and 2.3 years, respectively. When R0 resection was performed in patients without M1 diseases, 5-year survival rates
were 45% for patients without lymph node metastasis, and
50% for patients without lymph node metastasis nor portal
vein resection.

Selected Readings

Cherqui DC, Benoist S, Malassagne B, et al. (2000) Major liver resection for carcinoma in jaundiced patients without preoperative biliary drainage. Arch Surg 135:302–308

Ebata T, Nagino M, Kamiya J, et al. (2003) Hepatectomy with portal vein resection for hilar cholangiocarcinoma. Audit of 52 consecutive cases. Ann Surg 238:720–727

Kamiya S, Nagino M, Kanazawa H, et al. (2004) The value of bile replacement during external biliary drainage. An analysis of intestinal permeability, integrity, and microflora. Ann Surg 239:510–517

Kanazawa H, Nagino M, Kamiya S, et al. (2005) Synbiotics reduce postoperative infectious complications: a randomized controlled trial in biliary cancer patients undergoing hepatectomy. Langenbecks Arch Surg 390:104–113

Kitagawa Y, Nagino M, Kamiya J, et al. (2001) Lymph node metastasis from hilar cholangiocarcinoma: audit of 110 patients who underwent regional and paraaortic node dissection. Ann Surg 233:385–392

Nagino M, Kamiya J, Nishio H, et al. (2006) Two hundred forty consecutive portal vein embolizations before extended hepatectomy for biliary cancer. Surgical outcome and long-term follow-up. Ann Surg 243:364–372

Nimura Y, Hayakawa N, Kamiya J, et al. (1991) Combined portal vein and liver resection for carcinoma of the biliary tract. Br J Surg 78:727–731

Nimura Y, Hayakawa N, Kamiya J, et al. (1990) Hepatic segmentectomy with caudate lobe resection for bile duct carcinoma of the hepatic hilus. World J Surg 14:535–544

Nishio H, Nagino M, Nimura Y (2005) Surgical management of hilar cholangiocarcinoma: the Nagoya experience. HPB 7:259–262

Sugawara G, Nagino M, Nishio H, et al. (2006) Perioperative synbiotics treatment to prevent postoperative infectious complications in biliary cancer surgery. A randomized controlled trial. Ann Surg 244:706–714

20
Cancer of the Gallbladder

Xabier A. de Aretxabala and Ivan S. Roa

Pearls and Pitfalls

- Death related to gallbladder cancer is more common in countries where gallstones are prevalent.
- Almost all patients with gallbladder cancer have concomitant gallstones.
- Early-stage (T1) neoplasms may be undetected by the surgeon during the cholecystectomy, and thus pathologic examination of all cholecystectomy specimens is important.
- Perforation of the gallbladder during laparoscopic cholecystectomy in patients with incidental gallbladder carcinoma may account for the poor prognosis with minimally invasive approaches.
- Cholecystectomy alone is the appropriate surgical management of patients with invasion restricted to the mucosal (T0 or T1A lesions).
- Radical cholecystectomy (including lymphadenectomy and hepatic resection) is the recommended procedure for patients with tumor infiltrating the subserosal layer (T2 lesions).
- A complete microscopic and macroscopic negative resection (R0) is essential to avoid local recurrence and can achieve long-term survival.
- In countries with a high incidence of gallbladder cancer, careful screening and prophylactic cholecystectomy may be indicated in select patients.

K.I. Bland et al. (eds.), *Liver and Biliary Surgery*,
DOI 10.1007/978-1-84996-429-6_20,
© Springer-Verlag London Limited 2011

- Cholecystectomy is suggested for gallbladder polyps > 2 cm or when there are 3 or more polyps; polyps between 1 and 2 cm probably also warrant cholecystectomy in high risk regions.

Gallbladder cancer is considered a rare disease in many countries, yet in some countries, it represents one of the leading causes of cancer-related death; indeed, in Chile, gallbladder cancer is the leading cause of cancer-related death in women! This disease is common in certain geographic areas of the world, including Central and South America, Eastern Europe, northern India, and Japan.

Of all the risk factors associated with gallbladder cancer, gallstones are the most important. In fact, in Chile almost 95% of gallbladder cancers are associated with the presence of gallstones. Indeed, gallbladder carcinomas are found often in patients undergoing cholecystectomy for a presumably benign disease. The association of gallbladder carcinoma with gallstones may be related to chronic inflammatory changes in the mucosa incited by the presence of gallstones as well as an underlying genomic predisposition.

The inverse relation between the cholecystectomy rate and the incidence of gallbladder cancer reported by some authors further supports an association between gallstones and gallbladder cancer. This association is also apparent in Japan, where gallbladder cancer is associated with other entities such as the anomalous junction of the pancreatic and biliary ducts. Additional factors associated with gallbladder cancer include microcalcification of the gallbladder wall, carriers of salmonella typhae, and presumed but poorly understood environmental factors.

Symptoms

The majority of patients with early stages of gallbladder carcinoma are asymptomatic or have symptoms attributed to the presence of gallstones and not to the gallbladder carcinoma. Patients with clinically advanced gallbladder carcinoma present with symptoms or signs such as continuous

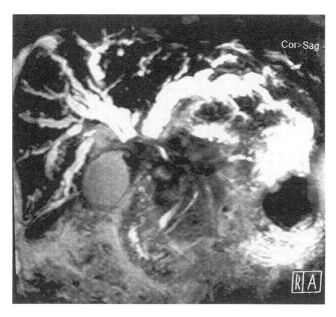

FIGURE 20.1. Typical image of a gallbladder tumor with invasion of the common bile duct.

abdominal pain, jaundice, anorexia, or a palpable mass. Jaundice, secondary to the obstruction of the common hepatic duct by direct tumor extension, is a common finding imparting a poor prognosis (Fig. 20.1).

Small, early-stage neoplasms are most frequently asymptomatic and are noted incidentally at cholecystectomy for cholelithiasis. Small, sessile neoplasms may go undetected during cholecystectomy or during gross examination of the resected specimen in up to 50% of patients. The sensitivity of ultrasonography and computed tomography (CT) in detecting these small lesions is low. Unfortunately, tumors readily detected by current imaging methods are frequently at an advanced stage where potentially curative intervention is unlikely (Fig. 20.2). Moreover, the existence of stones and inflammatory changes of the gallbladder wall that are common in the setting of gallbladder cancer further reduce the diagnostic accuracy of preoperative imaging.

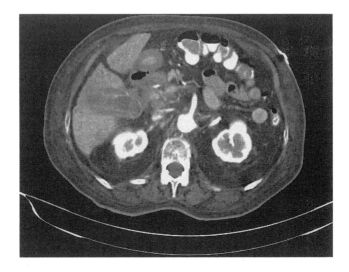

FIGURE 20.2. Computed tomography (CT) showing typical findings of an advanced gallbladder cancer. Stones are seen inside the gallbladder while liver infiltration is clearly observed.

The overall prognosis of patients with gallbladder cancer is poor, and 5-year survival in the more advanced neoplasms is rare. In areas with a high prevalence of gallstones, the detection of small, early-stage lesions may account for improved overall survival. In areas with a very high incidence of gallbladder cancer, involvement of the mucosa and/or limited muscular infiltration accounts for 20% of all gallbladder cancers. These patients have a 5-year survival rate greater than 75% when the lesion is noted in the cholecystectomy specimen and managed appropriately.

Classification

Historically, gallbladder cancer was classified according to the Nevin classification; however, this system had several shortcomings. First, it did not include those patients with invasion of the subserosal layer. Patients with infiltration of the subserosal layer represent the most important group among those with a resectable gallbladder cancer. This group is the largest and has an intermediate prognosis among those with gallbladder cancer. Second, the Nevin classification includes the cystic node, which is not always removed during routine cholecystectomy when gallbladder cancer is not suspected.

Currently, the most widely accepted staging system is the AJCC classification. This classification divides gallbladder cancers according to the depth of infiltration, adjacent organ involvement, lymph node involvement, and presence of metastases (Table 20.1). Thus, a preoperative search for these

TABLE 20.1. AJCC classification (TNM) of gallbladder cancer.

Primary tumor (T)

- TX: Primary tumor cannot be assessed

- T0: No evidence of primary tumor

- Tis: Carcinoma in situ

- T1: Tumor invades lamina propria or muscle layer

  ○ T1a: Tumor invades lamina propria

  ○ T1b: Tumor invades the muscle layer

- T2: Tumor invades the perimuscular connective tissue; no extension beyond the serosa or into the liver

- T3: Tumor perforates the serosa (visceral peritoneum) and/or directly invades the liver for <2 cm

- T4: Tumor invades into liver for >2 cm

Regional lymph nodes (N)

- NX: Regional lymph nodes cannot be assessed

- N0: No regional lymph node metastasis

- N1: Regional lymph node metastasis

Distant metastasis (M)

- MX: Distant metastasis cannot be assessed

- M0: No distant metastasis

- M1: Distant metastasis

potential findings proves to be important when selecting the appropriate treatment.

Preoperative Evaluation/Diagnosis

In patients in whom a preoperative diagnosis is possible, most have advanced-stage disease. These patients present generally with symptoms or signs such as jaundice, pain, and/or general malaise. Abdominal ultrasonography is usually the initial diagnostic procedure and may demonstrate dilation of the biliary tract, changes in the echogenicity of liver parenchyma, or a mass within the gallbladder (Fig. 20.3). CT and/or magnetic resonance imaging (MRI) are performed when gallbladder cancer is suspected to complete the staging and determine resectability. The use of tumor markers such as CEA and CA 19-9 has also been evaluated in the detection of early gallbladder cancer; however, the sensitivity and specificity of these tests in early-stage disease is low, and their value in screening for gallbladder cancer is unfounded.

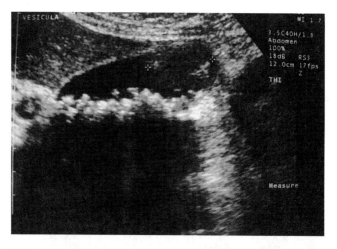

FIGURE 20.3. Gallbladder ultrasonography showing a mass compatible with a gallbladder cancer adjacent to the gallstones.

Differential diagnosis involves inflammatory and neoplastic disorders. The differential diagnosis includes cholangiocarcinoma, hepatocellular carcinoma, liver metastasis, and benign conditions such as benign gallbladder polyps or disorders related to gallstone disease, such as nonmobile gallstones, acute cholecystitis, and liver abscess.

Intraoperative Diagnosis

Intraoperative detection of gallbladder cancer is not unusual in countries where the incidence of gallbladder cancer is high. Completion of the resection in an attempt to achieve an R0 resection should be the primary goal under such conditions. Detailed abdominal exploration should be undertaken in a systematic approach including frozen section of potentially compromised distant areas. Presence of distant metastatic disease is a contraindication to proceed with radical cholecystectomy.

Where there is doubt about the depth of gallbladder wall involvement or when reliable frozen section analysis is not available, completion of the resection during a second operation after a detailed pathologic analysis of the specimen is a valid option. During the first operation, a thorough exploration should be performed to evaluate for metastatic disease, allowing more informative discussion with the patient and appropriate treatment planning.

Postoperative Diagnosis

A postoperative diagnosis may be made only after the gross and histologic examination of the specimen. Approximately 20% of the potentially curable gallbladder carcinomas are identified incidentally only on microscopic inspection. A thorough evaluation of the specimen is essential to determine the depth of invasion as well as the location in relation to the free wall of the gallbladder or adjacent to the liver bed. To facilitate the management of these tumors, these lesions are divided according to the depth and site of wall infiltration.

Treatment

Operative resection is the mainstay of treatment for resectable gallbladder cancer and offers the only opportunity for cure. The primary objective of the operation is to achieve an R0 resection. The extent of operative resection is dependent on the stage of the disease (Table 20.2). Thus, cholecystectomy alone is considered sufficient for Stage 0 and 1A lesions, whereas cholecystectomy with hepatectomy and hepatic hilar lymphadenectomy is indicated for stages IB through stage IV. Some groups even advocate pancreatoduodenal resection for the management of advanced gallbladder cancers, but results with such a radical resection remain controversial.

Mucosal infiltration. These neoplasms are usually detected on histopathologic examination of the cholecystectomy specimen.

TABLE 20.2. AJCC stage groupings.

Stage 0

- Tis, N0, M0

Stage IA

- T1A, N0, M0

Stage IB

- T1B, T2, N0, M0

Stage IIA

- T3, N0, M0

Stage IIB

- T1, N1, M0
- T2, N1, M0
- T3, N1, M0

Stage III

- T4, any N, M0

Stage IV

- Any T4, any N, M0

Simple cholecystectomy is sufficient for T1a or less disease. Five-year survival of this group of patients is 95%. Although there are descriptions of recurrence and mortality after cholecystectomy alone, these are extremely rare conditions that do not justify more aggressive resection.

Muscular invasion. When the gallbladder cancer invades the muscular layer of the wall of the gallbladder (T1b), the 5-year survival of these patients is less than for T1a lesions and is about 60%. As might be expected, the appropriate surgical treatment is controversial with the options of cholecystectomy alone and "extended" cholecystectomy, which includes wedge hepatic excision of the bed of the gallbladder combined with a locoregional lymphadenectomy; most series suggest better survival with a more aggressive, oncologic resection.

Subserosal invasion. Patients with infiltration of the subserosal layer represent 20% of all patients with gallbladder cancer. Unfortunately, the 5-year survival is only 40%. Although there is a lack of sufficient data, extended cholecystectomy is accepted as the gold standard in the treatment of these patients. Surgical intervention is indicated only after a complete evaluation to exclude distant metastases within the abdomen and thorax.

Radical extended cholecystectomy consists of a lymphadenectomy of the nodes along the hepatic pedicle, retropancreatic area, hepatic artery, and a wedge resection of the liver in the gallbladder bed. From a theoretic view, a pancreatoduodenal resection should be performed to eliminate the chance of nodal dissemination to the retropancreatic nodes in patients with choledochoduodenal lymph node invasion; however, the vastly greater morbidity of pancreatoduodenal resection must be balanced with the lower survival of these patients. Of the factors related to the prognosis, the presence of lymph node involvement is considered the most significant. The extent of the liver resection is also controversial and depends on operative findings and the surgeon's preference. A wide resection including segments V and IVb is performed; however, controlled trials evaluating advantages of a more extensive liver resection have not shown a convincing survival advantage.

Serosal invasion. Serosal infiltration (T3 disease) is associated with distant disease and poor survival (<20% 5-year survival). Serosal invasion is responsible for a much greater rate of peritoneal dissemination as well as a more extensive lymphatic dissemination. As a result, patients with serosal infiltration are less likely to present with resectable disease. The presence of findings such as involvement of the portal vein or hepatic artery or distant metastases (M disease), peritoneal dissemination, liver metastases, or distant nodal metastasis (paraaortic or celiac plexus) all preclude curative resection. Therefore, in these patients, a staging laparoscopy may be indicated before a formal celiotomy.

Operative Treatment

In summary, for stages 0 and IA (Table 20.3), most experts suggest that cholecystectomy alone is sufficient. For stages IB, IIA, and IIB, an aggressive radical extended cholecystectomy is indicated. For stages III, and IV, an extended cholecystectomy with lymphadenectomy (as for stages IIA and B) is standard of care, but many centers will also carry out a resection of the extrahepatic biliary tree and a right hepatectomy. If gallbladder cancer is suspected preoperatively, a staging laparoscopy before celiotomy is indicated because of the propensity of this aggressive disease to have hepatic or peritoneal metastases which might preclude any resection, although an argument might be made to resection the gallbladder if safe to prevent future complications and pain from an obstructed gallbladder secondary to tumor. When reoperating to "re-resect" a patient in whom the diagnosis was made after a recent laparoscopic cholecystectomy, many surgeons would also resect the trocar sites because of a somewhat increased incidence of trocar site implants of gallbladder cancer. Whether resection with an extended right trigesmentectomy, a pancreatoduodenectomy, and paraaortic lymphadenectomy offer benefit remains debatable. For M1 disease, resection is not indicated.

TABLE 20.3. Operative treatment of gallbladder cancer.

0, IA	Cholecystectomy alone
IA, IIA, IIB	Radical extended cholecystectomy
	– Resect previous trocar sites (if recent laparoscopic cholecystectomy)
	– Lymphadenectomy
	– Wedge hepatic excision of gallbladder bed
III, IV	Radical extended cholecystectomy
	– Resect previous trocar sites (if recent laparoscopic cholecystectomy)
	– Lymphadenectomy
	– Right hepatic lobectomy
	– Resection of extrahepatic biliary tree
	– Whether right trisegmentectomy, pancreatoduodenectomy, or para aortic lymphadenectomy adds benefit is uncertain

Prophylactic Cholecystectomy

With the aim of preventing the development of gallbladder cancer, prophylactic cholecystectomy may be a reasonable option in certain high-risk populations. In countries like Chile and Northern India where the disease has reached endemic proportions, cholecystectomy for gallstones should be considered even in asymptomatic patients. In fact, almost 20% of patients with gallbladder cancer had asymptomatic gallstone disease prior to the diagnosis of gallbladder cancer.

In countries or populations where the incidence of gallbladder cancer is high, analysis of factors, such as the possibility of developing gallbladder cancer (or symptomatic biliary colic) versus the postoperative morbidity and mortality of a cholecystectomy, shows that a cholecystectomy in patients with gallstones offers a cost-effective alternative in female patients more than 40 years old; at this age, the proportion of concomitant cancer is less than 2%, and the majority are

Tis or T1 lesions. In these high-risk populations, 60-year-old females with gallstones have as high as a 10% incidence of concomitant gallbladder cancer; note that many of the female population would have already undergone cholecystectomy. In contrast, among men, the incidence and correlation of gallstones and gallbladder cancer is less clear, and prophylactic cholecystectomy does not appear to be indicated.

Laparoscopic Cholecystectomy and Gallbladder Cancer

Since the introduction of laparoscopic cholecystectomy, numerous reports about the effect of a laparoscopic approach on the prognosis have been published. Recurrences at the trocar sites as a consequence of the minimally invasive approach have been reported. With more experience, however, it has been suggested that the approach itself is less likely to influence the prognosis than the related events that may occur during the laparoscopic approach, such as gallbladder perforation and bile leakage (extravasation of malignant cells). Although laparoscopic cholecystectomy should not be considered a factor associated with a poor prognosis, we must assume that gallbladder perforation and cancer cell exfoliation are responsible for a worse prognosis. Therefore, a meticulous technique must be carried out in all cases of laparoscopic cholecystectomy due to the possibility of an incidental gallbladder cancer. Probably more important is the concept that when a gallbladder cancer is suspected, we recommend conversion to an open procedure, but only if the surgeon is prepared to carry out an extended cholecystectomy if necessary.

Chemotherapy and Radiotherapy

Palliative chemotherapy. Because of the lower incidence of gallbladder cancer in developed countries where the majority of cancer research is performed, treatment protocols in gallbladder cancer are commonly extrapolated from studies of pancreatic and biliary tract neoplasms. During the 1980s and 1990s, 5-fluorouracil (5 FU) was the drug employed most commonly in the management of gallbladder cancer in both adjuvant and palliative settings. The results, however, were uniformly disappointing. Currently, chemotherapy with Gemcitabine or mitomycin C has demonstrated partial responses of up to 60%. The combination of cisplatin and Gemcitabine offers a new therapeutic alternative with higher responses than Gemcitabine alone. Capecitabine, another drug employed recently in the management of digestive cancers, has been tested in gallbladder cancer, as well, both with and without Gemcitabine.

Neoadjuvant therapy. The rationale for using chemoradiation in fully resected (Ro) gallbladder cancer is derived from experience in pancreas cancer that showed promising results. From a theoretic point of view, this treatment approach may have the advantages of reducing the implantability of cancer cells, allowing restaging later to identify those patients with progressive disease during the neoadjuvant treatment, and the concept that radiotherapy is more effective in well-oxygenated cells that have not been rendered hypoxic by a radical operation. With the above in mind, we designed a prospective, double-blind study comparing patients with potentially resectable gallbladder cancer who received chemoradiotherapy with 5 FU after the cholecystectomy and before performing the definitive reoperation with those patients not undergoing neoadjuvant treatment. This study did not show any benefit in resectability or survival; for patients undergoing chemoradiation, there was a considerable delay in the subsequent cholecystectomy due to a low platelet count which delayed operation.

Adjuvant therapy. The results of adjuvant chemoradiation therapy are equally discouraging. The ESPAC 1 trial, which analyzed the effect of both chemoradiotherapy and chemotherapy on the survival of patients having undergone a curative resection for pancreatic cancer, showed a significant benefit of only the chemotherapy arm. The main problem of this study was that 5 FU was the drug under analysis. At present, most authors are employing more effective drugs such as Gemcitabine and Capecitabine.

In gallbladder cancer, few studies have evaluated the role of adjuvant therapy. The main drawback of the above studies is the small number of patients and the lack of controlled studies. The Mayo Clinic reported a series of only 21 patients with completely resected gallbladder cancer who had a higher survival compared with historic controls. Duke University reported their experience in the management of 22 patients with resected gallbladder cancer who underwent external beam radiotherapy; this report advocates external beam radiotherapy with concomitant 5 FU in fully resected gallbladder cancers. Firm conclusions are difficult with such low numbers of patients. In our practice, we administer adjuvant therapy using capecitabine and radiation in patients with poor prognostic factors, such as positive lymph nodes and/or liver infiltration after resection.

Management of Jaundice

Due to the gallbladder's proximity to the bile duct, jaundice is a common finding in patients with advanced gallbladder cancer. Insertion of an endoscopic or percutaneous stent is a useful procedure to relieve symptoms caused by jaundice. Previous images of the biliary duct obtained by magnetic resonance are important in delineating the biliary anatomy. Analyzing the biliary tree will provide knowledge regarding the feasibility of drainage. Involvement of the segmented branches makes it difficult to drain the biliary tree completely, introducing the risk of cholangitis.

Special Situations

Gallbladder polyps. Most experts would suggest that a cholecystectomy is warranted for gallbladder polyps >1 cm but <2 cm even though the risk of gallbladder cancer is low. Polyps ≥ 2 cm or the presence of >3 polyps regardless of size should undergo cholecystectomy.

Porcelain gallbladder. The use of the term "porcelain gallbladder" can be confusing. In the past, many surgeons believed that a calcified gallbladder had a markedly increased risk (up to 10%) of harboring or predisposing to gallbladder cancer. The term "porcelain gallbladder" has, however, several forms. For the heavily calcified, thick-walled gallbladder evident on an abdominal radiograph, the risk of gallbladder cancer is really quite small; most surgeons would still recommend cholecystectomy, but the chance of gallbladder cancer is <2%. In contrast, when there are speckled areas of calcification in the mucosal layer, so-called milk of calcium, the association with cancer can be quite high (~10–15%) and warrants an aggressive approach with a very high suspicion of an underlying cancer.

Acknowledgments   Supported by Fondecyt Grant 1060375.

Selected Readings

American Joint Committee on Cancer (AJCC) (2002) Cancer Staging Manual. 6th edn. Springer, New York, pp. 139–144

De Aretxabala X, Roa I, Berrios M, et al. (2006) Chemoradiotherapy in gallbladder cancer. J Surg Oncol 93:699–704

De Aretxabala X, Roa I, Losada H, et al. (2006) Gallbladder cancer: an analysis of a series of 139 patients with invasion restricted to the subserosal layer. J Gastrointest Surg 10:186–192

Dixon E, Vollmer CM, Sahajpal A, et al. (2005) An aggressive surgical approach leads to improved survival in patients with gallbladder cancer. A 12-year study at a North American Center. Ann Surg 241:385–394

Fong Y, Jamagin W, Blumgart LH (2000) Gallbladder cancer: comparison of patients presenting initially for definitive operation with those presenting after prior noncurative intervention. Ann Surg 232:557–569

Stephen AE, Berger DL (2001) Carcinoma in the porcelain gallbladder: a relationship revisited. Surgery 129:699–703

Wakai T, Shirai Y, Yokoyama N, et al. (2003) Depth of subserosal invasion predicts long term survival after resection in patients with T2 gallbladder carcinoma. Ann Surg Oncol 10:447–454

Wistuba I, Gazdar AF (2004) Gallbladder cancer lessons from a rare tumor. Nature Review Cancer 4:695–706

Part V
Minimally Invasive Procedures

21
Laparoscopic Common Bile Duct Exploration

Leslie Karl Nathanson

Pearls and Pitfalls

- The majority of bile duct stones arise in the gallbladder and migrate down the cystic duct.
- Trans-cystic exploration clears successfully the bile duct (CBD) in 60–70% of patients; the remainder can be removed by post-operative endoscopic retrograde cholangiopancreatography (ERCP) or choledochotomy.
- This algorithm for bile duct stone management offers clinical benefit to 2/3 of patients and is 40% cheaper than selective use of pre-operative ERCP.
- Laparoscopic bile duct exploration skills need practice and team leadership in the operating room to be performed well but it will increase operating times.
- Primary duct stones require a drainage procedure as part of their management.

Basic Science

Secondary stones in the bile duct passed down through the cystic duct can be recognized by their facetted makeup, and are generally harder in consistency than primary bile duct stones. Primary bile duct stones tend to be a cast of the bile duct shape and fit together in that manner. Intra-operative

K.I. Bland et al. (eds.), *Liver and Biliary Surgery*,
DOI 10.1007/978-1-84996-429-6_21,
© Springer-Verlag London Limited 2011

cholangiography is the current gold standard for intra-operative bile duct stone identification during cholecystectomy, so these details need to be recognized to decide on the need for bilio-enteric duct drainage. In addition, note needs to be taken of the site of entry of the cystic duct, the bile duct diameter and the number, size and situation of the stones.

Clinical Presentation and Diagnosis

Two main methods of managing bile duct stones have emerged.

Laparoscopic cholecystectomy is undertaken following pre-operative clearance of CBD stones using ERCP selectively based on judicious use of MRI or CT Cholangiography. A useful clinical risk algorithm (Table 21.1) prior to cholecystectomy, stratifies patients into 4 risk groups for CBD stones. This is based on clinical signs, serum bilirubin levels, liver function tests (LFTs), serum lipase and the presence or absence of a dilated bile duct on ultrasound (US). The very high risk group for stones (93%) should undergo ERCP as the next step. The high risk (34%) group proceeds to MRI

TABLE 21.1. The toolbox.

A well informed team

Second camera and stack

Cholangiogram catheter

C-arm fluoroscopy

Exploration catheter with dormia basket and side arm for x-ray contrast injection

3 and 5 mm flexible choledochoscopes

Rigid ureteroscope

Lithoclast and spark gap lithotripsy

Antegrade bile duct stents and laparoscopic introducers

T-tubes

or CT cholangiography with ERCP being performed only for those patients with confirmed stones. The low (4%) risk group require no further preoperative investigation but should have an operative cholangiogram. Those patients in the very low (<1%) risk group have no need for a cholangiogram to detect CBD stones.

The second approach to bile duct stones is the one I would like to expand on in this chapter. Preoperative investigations are confined to US, serum LFTs and serum lipase. ERCP is reserved only for patients presenting with severe cholangitis or pancreatitis. Operative cholangiography forms the basis for detecting stones and decisions on how to clear them. The clinical benefits for 70% of patients are the use of a single stage procedure, avoidance of either sphincterotomy or choledochotomy, rapid post operative recovery and substantial overall cost savings.

Operative Techniques

Standard exposure is initiated with umbilical and three subcostal ports. During dissection of the cystic duct its size is noted and dissection taken down closer to the common hepatic duct to avoid spiral valves. The cystic duct course into the CBD (direct, into the right hepatic duct, or very low down near the ampulla), CBD diameter, coupled with the size, shape and number of bile duct stones are all noted during the cholangiography (Fig. 21.1a). This is performed using an end hole 4F ureteric catheter under fluoroscopic imaging. If there is uncertainty in interpreting the images, it may be helpful to wash contrast out with saline and to re-run the cholangiogram. Imaging during the washout phase can be as helpful as during the contrast run to demonstrate details of the stones.

The mainstay for stone extraction in most patients is fluoroscopic guided stone trapping baskets deployed through the Olsen-Reddick cholangiogram clamp which has an inner working diameter of 6F (Fig. 21.1b). It is also used to deploy the Fogarty balloon catheter and therefore facilitates quick exchanges of stone extraction equipment.

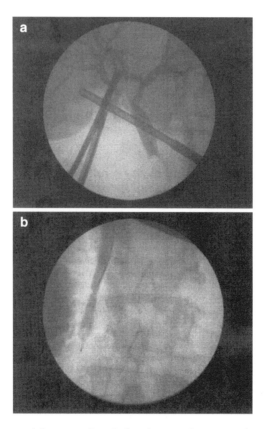

FIGURE 21.1. (**a**) composite cholangiogram demonstrating a filling defect at lower end of common bile duct. (**b**) Fluoroscopic view of bile duct showing a four-wire basket retrieving a lower common bile duct stone (Reprinted from Nathanson and Shaw, 2005. Copyright 2005. With permission from Elsevier).

Trans-Cystic Stone Extraction

Once bile ducts are confirmed and considered suitable for trans-cystic extraction the 4F cholangiogram catheter is exchanged for the 5.5F catheter with injection side arm and dormia basket. Patients considered at high risk of bile duct stones (Table 21.1), may have some time saved by using the larger catheter for the diagnostic cholangiogram.

The *catheter tip* is advanced to the first stone, its tip placed just beyond the stone and then the dormia basket extended down the catheter. Once the tip of the dormia starts emerging from the catheter, judged by fluoroscopic monitoring, the dormia basket position is held steady and the catheter withdrawn, to allow the basket to deploy around the stone. Engagement of the wires around the stone can be encouraged by a gentle vibrating motion of the basket, which with the captured stone is then withdrawn slowly out of the cystic duct. The stone is placed in a suitable area in the abdominal cavity for later removal with the gallbladder. This process is repeated in sequence, working down toward the ampulla. Concerns are often raised about the need for cystic duct dilation to allow stone extraction. In practice this is seldom a problem, because secondary stones by definition have migrated down the cystic duct and will with gentle persuasion can be retrieved and withdrawn the other way. Obviously, common sense is required when assessing the relative diameter of the stone and cystic duct and alternate clearance used when gross disparity exists.

The identification of stones in the biliary tree proximal to the cystic duct entry on initial cholangiography may be a reason to choose either choledochotomy, or ERCP clearance. Before a decision is made, a number of helpful steps should be considered. Firstly, on rare occasions the basket can be deployed upwards from the cystic duct. Secondly streaming the stones from the proximal CHD into the distal bile duct can often be achieved. Angulation of the operating table to a head down and right side down position, alters bile duct orientation. This, coupled with instrumental agitation of the liver, followed by gentle stroking of the extra-hepatic bile duct toward the ampulla, frequently encourages bile flow towards the ampulla, often surprisingly dislodging stones which float upwards and distally. However, multiple proximally located stones may make this less successful.

On occasions, calculi will come out in a fragmented fashion. In this instance, if doubt exists regarding completeness of stone clearance when observing the check cholangiogram, often in the presence of a dilated duct, further visual inspection with a small caliber flexible choledochoscope is helpful.

Care must be taken near the distal common duct not to deploy the basket in the ampulla since this may cause its mucosa to become jammed in the dormia basket wires. A clue to this problem is found when there is rather more early resistance than expected to withdrawal of the dormia basket, and fluoroscopic inversion of the ampulla and distal bile duct occurs. *The urge to continue withdrawal of the catheter should be resisted.* Disentanglement of the ampulla mucosa in the basket is easily achieved by simply pushing the basket and catheter into the duodenum, until the tip of the catheter is in the duodenum. The basket is then withdrawn into the catheter, which is, in turn, withdrawn back into the bile duct. Avoidance of this trauma to the ampulla will minimize the risk of inducing acute pancreatitis or long term ampullary scarring.

A stone impacted in the ampulla requires a number of strategies. A considerable amount of time can be wasted persisting with one technique rather than moving on to use others. For an apparently impacted stone, the first step is to pass a 5F Fogarty balloon catheter past the stone, to inflate the balloon sufficient to retrieve it and then by traction displace the stone. Once the stone is dislodged sufficiently to allow contrast to flow past it, dormia basket retrieval is preferred, as ongoing balloon extraction runs the risk of displacing the stone into the proximal bile ducts. This maneuver most often fails because the Fogarty balloon catheter cannot be negotiated past the stone. The next step is the use of lithotripsy. The easiest access is to use a flexible choledochoscope and a Calcutript catheter is used to break up the stone once it is in view. This is done only enough to crack the stone into large fragments and this then allows the process to be completed by basket retrieval. Great care must be taken to avoid misdirecting the Calcutript onto the bile duct wall as this will result in bile duct perforation. The tip of the choledochoscope is also at risk of damage if activation occurs within it.

An alternative approach is to cannulate the cystic duct with a rigid ureteroscope. This is inserted via the most lateral subcostal port and is surprisingly easy to use. The distal bile duct and stone on view allows use of the LithoClast which is remarkably quick and safe at achieving stone disruption but can only be used through a rigid scope.

Following CBD exploration, decompression of the bile duct is only advocated after removal of severely impacted stones or for patients with significant cholangitis or who have required significant manipulation around the ampulla. The choice for decompression is an antegrade 7F Cotton-Leung stent placed across the ampulla, or a "C" tube placed in the cystic duct, held in place with a ligature and exteriorized.

Cystic duct closure should be with a clip adequate for its diameter or by means of an Endoloop. A sub-hepatic drain is used selectively after trans-cystic stone clearance.

Choledochotomy

Choledochotomy is reserved for situations where trans-cystic access is unsuitable, stone load is excessive or if stones are situated proximally. It should be avoided in ducts less than 8 mm diameter as assessed by operative cholangiography due to the unacceptable risk of bile duct stricture.

A supra-duodenal longitudinal choledochotomy is made with sharp scissors and sparing diathermy. "Stay" sutures to the margin of the opening are not useful as they interfere with the operative field. Initial clearance is by irrigation into the choledochotomy using the standard suction/irrigator with the resultant fluid backflow from the choledochotomy depositing stones into the subhepatic pouch. A 5 mm flexible choledochoscope with an adequate instrument channel is guided down a port and explores the proximal and distal duct systems to enable basket removal of stones under vision. The techniques for managing impacted stones are identical to those described for the trans-cystic exploration. A final check cholangiogram is performed using the Olsen-Reddick clamp. Contrast is injected first for fluoroscopic imaging of the proximal bile duct and then to outline the distal bile duct when the clamp is re-applied.

Primary closure is performed unless considerable manipulation in the area of the ampulla was required, or severe cholangitis was present. A fine monofilament suture should be placed with small neat bites of bile duct wall to minimize narrowing the duct. An access port in the left upper quadrant may provide improved ergonomics for manipulating the needle holder and should be added without hesitation if required.

Bile duct decompression can be achieved with a "T" tube, a stent placed through the sphincter of Oddi, or by means of a "C" tube. The "T" tube selected is usually the largest that will fit comfortably in the bile duct. Once it is introduced via one of the ports and positioned, the bile duct is sutured with a monofilament absorbable suture. The end of the tube is exteriorized in the most direct way to the skin. To document duct stone clearance in the post-operative phase, contrast imaging through the T-tube may be at day 4, or later according to personal preference. However removal of the "T" tube should be delayed until at least 4 weeks because the extent of inflammatory "walling off" of the tract is less after laparoscopy than open surgery and bile leak more common with earlier T-Tube removal.

The antegrade insertion of a 7F Cotton-Leung plastic stent is a useful alternative. Care must be taken by either fluoroscopy or choledochoscopy to ensure that the stent straddles the ampulla correctly. It will require endoscopic removal a month later.

The "C" tube is a tube drain that can be placed via the cystic duct (see above). A subhepatic closed low pressure suction drain is always placed after choledochotomy.

Primary Duct Stones

For patient with clear evidence of primary duct stones, a biliary drainage procedure is required. This may be by endo-scopic sphincterotomy, choledocho-jejunostomy Roux-en-Y or choledochoduodenostomy. In situations where choledo-chotomy is cannot be performed, then clearance of the bile duct and drainage by endoscopic retrograde cholangiography and sphincterotomy seems reasonable. In older patients, choledochotomy clearance may be considered and achieved in much the same way as at open surgery, by suture of the opened duct to the duodenum to form a choledochoduode-nostomy. Planning for this should start at the time of chole-dochotomy so that the incision is made close to the duodenum, which will then lie comfortably after completion of the anas-tomosis. For younger patients the risks of bile duct "sump syndrome" developing over many years mandate that a retrocolic Roux-en-Y bypass provides the best outcome. This can be achieved by laparoscopic means, but if it is not proceeding smoothly should be completed as an open procedure.

Outcomes

To date experience with laparoscopic bile duct clearance has accumulated slowly. The benefits for patients of trans-cystic stone clearance, with hospital discharge within a day or two of surgery, and avoidance of choledochotomy and drainage tubes has been under appreciated. Review of the data on trans-cystic approaches in all of the randomized studies to date show benefit in terms of operative time and hospital stay, but have tended to be analyzed as a single group with those patients having choledochotomy. However, trans-cystic exploration does require careful co-ordination of staff and of available equipment in the operating rooms, is not always predictable and requires frequent changes in strategy. This entails the surgeon assuming the role of pre-planning and leadership and as staff confidence and efficiency in the techniques is attained, the clinical and cost benefits will begin to be appreciated. The use of cholangiography in selecting out patients with stones is simple and has the added benefit of confirming biliary anatomy during cholecystectomy. Failed trans-cystic exploration will occur in 20–30% of patients, with the choices for stone clearance then being laparoscopic choledochotomy, open choledochotomy or post-operative ERCP. The only randomized trial of this choice suggests that the clinical outcome is similar for laparoscopic choledochotomy and postoperative ERCP. This therefore requires other factors to be considered in achieving an appropriate management decision, such as the need for patient transfer, long delays for treatment, surgical experience and patient preference.

Cost as an issue is notoriously difficult to factor into the choice of management. Since 2000, data have suggested that laparoscopic bile duct clearance costs less than half that of pre-operative ERCP clearance. Urbach et al looked at the problem from a different perspective, showing that the cost per residual bile duct stone is 50 times less. Yet we have not seen a shift in clinical practice. This may be due to the more recent selective use of pre-operative ERCP imaging, and the difficulty most clinicians have in trusting systems of cost analys is sufficiently to outweigh clinical factors. For this reason a somewhat simple analysis of cost will be used as an illustration.

As discussed earlier the two approaches of selective pre-operative ERCP clearance or trans-cystic exploration and post-operative ERCP seem reasonable ways to remove bile duct stones. Lui et al. have outlined a system of clinical factor analysis (Table 21.2) to use pre-operative ERCP most efficiently. This divides patients into four groups at risk of having bile duct stones each managed differently. The very high risk group goes straight to ERCP, patients in the high risk group undergo MRI imaging to select out those needing ERCP, the low risk group have an operative cholangiogram only, and the very low risk group have no cholangiogram at all.

TABLE 21.2. System for patient selection for the selective use of imaging to maximize pre-operative ERCP as a therapeutic procedure (Data from Liu et al., 2001).

Total 440 patients	Group 1 (27)	Group 2 (37)	Group 3 (52)	Group 4 (324)
Symptoms	No gallbladder tenderness	Tender gallbladder	Tender gallbladder	Tender/non tender gallbladder
US CBD Diam	≥ 5 mm	≥ 5 mm	<5 mm	<5 mm
Bilirubin ≥ 25 μmol/l				
Alk. phos ≥ 150 U/l	Presence of ≥ 2 of these serum values	Presence of ≥ 2 of these serum values	Presence of ≥ 2 of these serum values	None of these values abnormal
AST ≥ 100 U/l				
ALT ≥ 100 U/l				
Lipase	Normal	May be elevated	May be elevated	Normal
Risk CBD stones	93%	32%	4%	<1%
Management	Pre-op. ERCP + cholangiogram	MRCP ± Pre-op. ERCP + cholangiogram	Cholangiogram	No cholangiogram

An estimate of procedural costs can be made using these data. The number and type of procedure is taken directly from Table 21.3. This exercise values the costs of the various components added to cholecystectomy as: MRI $800, cholangiogram $400, ERCP clearance $4000, and trans-cystic clearance $1000.

The costs can be compared (Table 21.3) using the same data employing a selective cholangiography policy, the ability to clear 2/3 patients trans-cystically with post-operative ERCP for the remainder. This illustrates a 40% cost saving for laparoscopic exploration. The exercise also lends itself to

TABLE 21.3. Costs added to laparoscopic cholecystectomy comparing selected use of pre-operative ERCP and laparoscopic clearance for group 1, 2, 3 (116 patients out of 440), 40 of whom have bile duct stones (Data from Liu et al., 2001).

	Refined use of pre-op ERCP		Laparoscopic CBD clearance and post-op ERCP		
Pre-op ERCP	36				
		$144,000			
MRI	37				
		$29,600			
Cholangiogram	116				
		$46,400			
			116		Cholangiogram
				$46 400	
			27		Trans-cystic clearance
				$27 000	
			13		Post-op ERCP
				$52 000	
Total cost		$220 000		$125 400	

recalculation by surgeons in various parts of the world with differing medical systems and cost considerations.

In summary, laparoscopic bile duct exploration simplifies pre-operative investigations to US and LFTs. Two of very three patients will avoid choledochotomy or ERCP with this approach which provides the patient a one stage procedure to solve their problem and results in cost savings of 40%.

There may also be benefit of a lower incidence of ampullary strictures in the long term. Although this is an area for which there are little data, the clinical benefits of avoiding potential ERCP sphincter damage and late re-stenosis (reported in up to 20% of patients followed for 20 years), may only become apparent after many years.

For these reasons it is my view that the clinical and cost benefits should persuade biliary surgeons to develop their skills of laparoscopic bile duct clearance. Performance should be monitored by constant audit of outcome. If this does not match the outcomes of the published trials, further training should be sought to develop the expertise. This applies equally in my view to high and low volume surgeons.

Selected Readings

Cuschieri A, Lezoche E, Mornino M, et al. (1999) E.A.E.S. multicenter prospective randomized trial comparing two-stage vs single-stage management of patients with gallstone disease and ductal calculi. Surgical Endoscopy 13:952–957

Liu TH, Consorti ET, Kawashima A, et al. (2001) Patient evaluation with selective use of magnetic resonance cholangiography and endoscopic retrograde cholangiopancreatography before laparoscopic cholecystectomy. Ann Surg 234:33–40

Nathanson LK, Shaw IM (2005) Gallstones. In: Garden OJ (ed) Hepatobiliary and pancreatic surgery, 3rd edn. Elsevier, London, p 181

Nathanson LK, O'Rourke NA, Martin IJ, et al. (2005) Post-operative ERCP versus laparoscopic choledochotomy for clearance of selected bile duct calculi: a randomized trial. Ann Surg 242:188–192

Rhodes M, Sussman L, Cohen L, Lewis MP (1998) Randomised trial of laparoscopic exploration of common bile duct versus postoperative endoscopic retrograde cholangiography for common bile duct stones. Lancet 351:159–161

Sgourakis G, Karaliotas K (2002) Laparoscopic common bile duct exploration and cholecystectomy versus endoscopic stone extraction and laparoscopic cholecystectomy for choledocholithiasis. A prospective randomized study. Minerva Chirurgica 57:467–474

Traverso LW (2000) A cost analysis of the treatment of common bile duct stones discovered during cholecystectomy. Semin Laparosc Surg 7:302–307

Urbach DR, Khanjanchee YS, Jobe BA, et al. (2001) Cost-effective management of common bile duct stones. Surg Endosc 15:4–13

Index

A
Absolute risk, 41–42
Adjuvant therapy, 84, 105–108
Angiosarcomas, 231, 236
Axillary dissection, 17, 24, 31, 32, 36
Axillary surgery, 96, 98, 99

B
Basal cell carcinoma, 164–166
Biopsy, 211, 212, 214–215, 220–221, 236, 238
Brachytherapy, 240–241
Breast, 61–81
Breast cancer, 17–22, 24–37, 61–67, 71, 78–81, 127–132, 134, 135, 138–140, 142–144
Breast conservation, 21, 29, 30
Breast mass, 3, 5, 6
Breast pain, 3, 4, 6, 9
Breast reconstruction, 101–104, 147–153

C
Carcinoma, 61–81
Chemotherapy, 17, 18, 23, 25, 33, 34, 36, 113, 117–124, 230, 240, 242–245
Core biopsy, 87, 89, 96

D
Diagnosis, 199–202, 206–208
Ductal, 61–81

E
Early breast cancer, 91, 105, 106, 108, 109
Endocrine therapy, 113, 117–119, 122, 124
Estrogen receptor, 128, 130
Excision margin, 201, 203

F
Family history, 39–59
Follow-up, 208–209

H
Hereditary cancer, 53, 57
High risk, 39–59
Hormone therapy, 17

I
Implant breast reconstruction, 149–151
In-transit melanoma, 223
Indicators, 39–59
Inflammatory breast cancer, 113, 115, 122–124

L

Lifetime risk, 40, 42
Lobular origin, 61–81
Locally advanced breast cancer,
    113–124

M

Mammography, 88, 111
Mastectomy, 17, 23, 25, 29–31, 36,
    83, 84, 93–95, 98, 99,
    101–104, 109–111
Melanoma, 159, 162, 166–169,
    171–197, 199–227
Metastasectomy, 212, 224, 225
Metastatic, 127–144
Microscopic lesions, 39–59

N

Neoadjuvant, 18, 23, 34
Neoadjuvant therapy, 84, 100,
    109–110
Nipple discharge, 6, 14
Nipple-areola reconstruction, 151,
    153, 154

P

Personal history, 44, 54
Pigmented lesions, 159, 162,
    167, 168
Progesterone receptor, 128, 130
Punch biopsy, 160, 161, 168

R

Radiation, 17, 19, 21, 23, 24, 29, 31,
    33, 34, 36

Radiation therapy, 230, 231, 238,
    240–242
Reconstruction, 17, 30

S

Sarcomas, 229–245
Selective sentinel lymphadenec-
    tomy (SSL), 199, 200,
    204–206, 209, 210
Sentinel lymph node, 189–197,
    212, 220–222, 226
Sentinel lymph node biopsy,
    17, 32
Sentinel node, 171, 172, 178,
    182–184, 186
Sentinel node biopsy, 97
Skin cancer, 191
Skin lesions, 159–169
Skin-sparing, 17, 29, 30
Soft tissue, 229–245
Squamous cell carcinoma,
    163–166
Staging, 171–188, 199, 202–204,
    206, 232–235, 237, 242, 245
Surgical complications, 209–210

T

Transverse rectus abdominus
    myocutaneous (TRAM)
    flap, 150, 152, 153
Trastuzumab, 113, 121, 123, 124
Treatment, 129–132, 135, 139,
    142–144

W

Wide local excision, 216

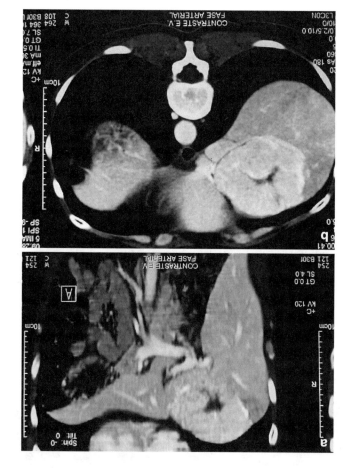

FIGURE 3.4. (**a, b**) CTs of focal nodular hyperplasia showing the typical central radial scar.

Treatment of known FNH is limited to observational surveillance and discontinuation of oral contraceptives in women. Because there is no worry of malignant degeneration or other complications within the lesion (bleeding, necrosis, abscess, etc.), there is no justification for resection unless there are symptoms related to its mass effect. Under these circumstances, the operative treatment consists of enucleation; there is no need to perform a wedge-type excision or formal

anatomic resection of a known FNH. The vast majority of FNHs, however, are resected because of an uncertain diagnosis; in these cases, the resection is performed according to location and with oncologic intent.

Hepatocellular Adenoma

Hepatocellular adenomas (HA) are usually seen in young women and are associated with the use of hormones. These benign neoplasms are well-delineated, solitary, benign neoplasms of a few centimeters in size, yellow-pink in color, soft on palpation, and showing foci of hemorrhagic dots on the transected surface. Certain patient populations are predisposed to developing HA, including patients with galactosemia, type 1 glycogen deposits, Turner's and Klinefelter's syndromes, and most conspicuously, users of oral contraceptives, estrogens, androgens, danazol, clomiphene, and growth hormone. The relationship between HA and oral contraceptives, as well as with pregnancy, is well-described; indeed, patients showing growth of an HA during pregnancy are well-documented, lending strong support to the association of HA and steroid sex hormones. A decrease in the size of the HA has also been described when oral contraceptives are discontinued.

The risk of developing HA in oral contraceptive users depends on the concentration of the estrogen, duration of use (more than 2 years), and the woman's age (>30 years of age). Overall, however, the risk is extremely low and must vary with individual genomic predisposition. Of concern, however, is that there is a greater risk of rupture and bleeding during pregnancy in patients with known HA. In addition, the co-existence of HA and the development of hepatocellular carcinoma has been postulated, although the evidence supporting a definite association is difficult to confirm. Histologically, HAs consist of a homogeneous population of hepatocytes that may contain abundant glycogen; a notable absence of the portal triads and biliary ducts and

the presence of thin-walled blood vessels and peliosis are pathognomonic findings. Sometimes it can be very difficult to differentiate well-differentiated hepatocarcinomas from HAs.

Adenomas are usually asymptomatic but on rare occasions may present with rupture and massive bleeding. They are most often detected on imaging studies performed for other, non-specific abdominal symptoms that are difficult to relate to the lesion. Laboratory work-up for abnormalities in liver enzymes, tumor markers, or viral infection should be normal. Imaging studies are crucial for their categorization to differentiate HAs from FNH, hepatocellular carcinoma, or metastases; a scintigraphic study (with ^{99m}Tc colloid sulphur), as described previously in the differential diagnosis with FNH, may be useful. On US, HA appears as an echogenic lesion. On CT, it looks hyperdense prior to giving intravenous contrast and variable in intensity after contrast administration. On MRI, the HA is hyperintense on T1-weighted images, iso-intense or less prominent on T2-weighted images, and with the use of gadolinium, it becomes very prominent. Angiography is indicated rarely but will show a hypervascularized lesion with areas of hemorrhage and tortuous vessels. The diagnosis of HA is made usually by excluding other alternatives more pathognomonic on imaging. Differentiation from hepatocellular carcinoma is most problematic and may require resection to prove. Biopsy of the lesion, as mentioned in the description of FNH, is not indicated, because it is not helpful.

The appropriate treatment of HA is resection when there is risk of rupture, bleeding, or question of the diagnosis. The operative approach, laparotomy or laparoscopy, will depend on the location and characteristics of the lesion. Enucleation, wedge resection, or local ablation is usually sufficient. Although experience with alcohol injection or radiofrequency ablation is limited, these approaches seem reasonable in selected situations. Oral contraceptives must be stopped, and long-term follow-up with ultrasonography is recommended in patients in whom resection is not indicated.

Angiomyolipoma

This rare, benign neoplasm of mesenchymal origin is usually seen in the kidney but also rarely in the liver. Its relationship to tuberous sclerosis is not well-defined but appears to be real. The histologic characteristics consist of a mixture of lipomatous tissue, blood vessels, and smooth muscle in variable proportions. The tumor may be single or multiple and often reaches quite a large size. The pre-operative diagnosis can be difficult, but the MRI finding of a tumor full of fat is useful for diagnosis. Percutaneous biopsy has a poor

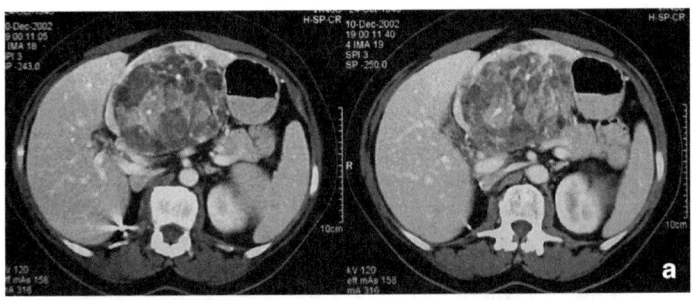

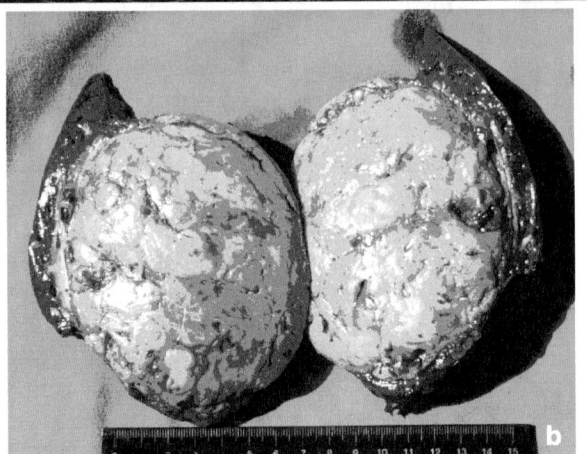

FIGURE 3.5. Angiomyolipoma. (**a**) CT demonstrating a vascular lesion with fatty infiltration. (**b**) Cut surface of resected neoplasm.

yield and may suggest a sarcoma. The malignant potential of this tumor is not clear. Given the rarity of this neoplasm and its diagnostic difficulty, it seems prudent to recommend resection (Fig. 3.5a, b).

Inflammatory Pseudotumor of the Liver

This entity was described in the liver in 1953. This lesion presents as a well-defined mass with foci of hemorrhage and necrosis, a chronic inflammatory infiltrate, and proliferation of fibrous elements. Although often treated aggressively by resection, its natural evolution when diagnosed correctly is toward spontaneous regression. The pathogenesis has been attributed to an infectious origin with an intense inflammatory response; others have treated inflammatory pseudotumors with steroids. The diagnosis is based ultimately on the histology, and if suspected highly, a biopsy would preclude resection; however, as with all liver tumors, biopsy is fraught with the possibility of seeding if the tumor is malignant, and this possibility should be kept in mind when considering biopsy. Because of such concerns, resection is the usual approach to these unusual liver tumors.

Other Benign Tumors

There is a variety of other benign neoplasms in the liver, but each has an extremely low incidence, including biliary hamartoma, solitary fibrous tumor, benign mesothelioma, lipoma associated with myolipoma or angiolipoma, mesenchymal hamartoma, mixoma, and teratoma.

Incidentally Discovered Liver Lesions

With the widespread use of state-of-the-art imaging, the recognition of liver lesions has become relatively frequent. These abnormalities on imaging can cause great anxiety in

the patient, and the clinician must present an organized, systematic approach to diagnosis and therapy. The first point is to differentiate cystic from solid lesions (see Chapter 2). Once a cystic lesion has been excluded, the next step is to determine whether this solid tumor is benign or malignant, because this may determine either resection versus observation or enucleation versus formal, anatomic resection. The patient's age, history, and clinical background becomes very important. The presence of other hepatic diseases, history of extrahepatic malignancies, neoplasias that could have given rise to a metastasis, alcoholism, trauma, viral infections, particularly hepatitis B or C, and the use of medications, mainly estrogens, contraceptives, or toxic drugs, may prove very important. Laboratory evaluation usually includes hepatic function tests and screening for the existence of markers of past or current hepatitis B or C infection. Tumor markers such as α fetoprotein and embryonic antigen are used selectively, based on the clinical history and characteristics of imaging. Imaging studies usually begin with US, but usually also require CT and/or MRI to make a more definitive diagnosis. Biliary scintigraphy may differentiate adenoma from focal nodular hyperplasia. Selective arteriography is used or indicated only infrequently but may be helpful to detect neovasculature characteristic of hepatocellular carcinoma.

In summary, the most common benign tumors of the liver are cavernous hemangioma, hepato-cellular adenoma (HA), and focal nodular hyperplasia (FNH). Imaging studies usually allow a confident diagnosis of these three benign lesions. When there is question of the diagnosis, resection is usually indicated, because percutaneous liver biopsy risks seeding of the neoplasm if malignant. When the diagnosis is HA, we usually recommend resection, because HA is associated with the risk of bleeding, rupture, or potential malignant degeneration. Hemangiomas and FNH are managed by observation and have a operative indication only if they are symptomatic.

Small lesions (<2 cm) are difficult to characterize with imaging, and if there are no risk factors for neoplasia, we recommend a program of periodic surveillance, particularly if

the lesion is difficult to access surgically. If the lesion increases in size, resection is usually necessary.

Selected Readings

Farges O, Daradkeh S, Bismuth H (1995) Cavernous hemangiomas of the liver: are there any indications for resection? World J Surg 19:19–24

Hoffman AL, Emre S, Verham RP, et al. (1997) Hepatic – angiomyolipoma: two case reports of caudate-based lesions and review of the literature. Liver Transpl Surg 3:46–53

Koea J, Broadhurst G, Rodgers M, McCall J (2003) Inflammatory pseudotumor of the liver: demographics, diagnosis and the case for nonoperative management. J Am Coll Surg 196:226–235

Kuo PC, Lewis WD, Jenkins RL (1994) Treatment of giant liver hemangiomas of the liver by enucleation. J Am Coll Surg 178:49–53

Nagorney DM (1995) Benign hepatic tumors: focal nodular hyperplasia and hepatocellular adenoma. World J Surg 19:13–18

Roocks JB, Ory HW, Ishak KG, et al. (1979) Epidemiology of hepatocellular adenoma. The role of oral contraceptive use. JAMA 242:644–648

Weimann A, Ringe B, Klempnauer J, et al. (1997) Benign liver tumors: differential diagnosis and indications for surgery. World J Surg 21:983–991

4
Hepatic Abscess: Current Concepts

Sanchez M. William and Hernando O. Abaunza

Pearls and Pitfalls

- Due to its dual circulation, the liver has a greater probability of developing abscesses of metastatic bacterial origin from other tissues.
- Over the past 30 years, the incidence of pyogenic liver abscess has increased, and the etiologies have changed.
- Risk factors for developing pyogenic liver abscesses include transplant patients, mainly liver transplants, immunosuppressive diseases, cancer, diabetes, biliary diseases, and other nonspecific conditions such as old age, alcoholism, and the presence of infectious gastrointestinal diseases.
- Hospital mortality is increased in patients with pyogenic liver abscesses in the presence of cancer, hyperbilirubinemia, leukocytosis (>20,000 cells/mm^3), hypoalbuminemia, pleural effusion, intraperitoneal perforation of an abdominal viscus, multiple small abscesses, and diabetes.
- Signs and symptoms are usually non-specific and are related to the local and systemic response to the infection.
- Treatment of pyogenic liver abscesses includes one or more of the following modalities: (1) antibiotic therapy, (2) percutaneous drainage, (3) operative drainage, and (4) hepatic resection.

K.I. Bland et al. (eds.), *Liver and Biliary Surgery*,
DOI 10.1007/978-1-84996-429-6_4,
© Springer-Verlag London Limited 2011

- Current management of pyogenic liver abscesses involves drainage under image guidance.
- Amebic liver abscesses are more common in males than in females, are found rarely in children, and are usually present in young individuals with an incidence greater during the summer months in endemic areas. About 80% of amoebic abscesses present as a solitary lesion localized in the right lobe.
- Unlike pyogenic abscesses, amoebic abscesses present in a more subacute manner often with symptoms for weeks or even months.
- Serum antibodies, especially IgG, offer value (70–90%) for the diagnosis of amoebic liver abscesses.
- Treatment for amoebic liver abscess is based on therapy with metronidazole; success rates range from 40% to 90%.

Introduction

Hippocrates described liver abscesses and suggested that the nature of the drainage used could change the prognosis of this disease. In 1836, John Bright described the clinicopathologic manifestations, but it was Ochsner in 1938 who published his classic review of 47 patients, noting a mortality of 80%.

Because of its dual circulation, the liver has a greater probability of developing "metastatic" abscesses of hematogenous origin secondary to infections originating in other tissues. Traditionally, three types of liver abscesses have been described: pyogenic, amoebic, and hydatid. In the current world literature, there are reports of liver abscesses secondary to many of types of bacteria, fungi, and parasites. This chapter focuses on pyogenic and amoebic abscesses, because they account for more than 90% of all liver abscesses.

Pyogenic Abscess

Incidence: During the past 30 years, the incidence of pyogenic abscesses has increased in certain patient populations. The widespread use of hepatic ultrasonography and

other modalities of non-invasive imaging has been an important contributing factor to the increase in the number of cases diagnosed and, therefore, in part to its greater incidence.

Other factors associated with this rise in incidence include the increasing use of chemotherapy for malignancies, immunosuppressive agents for organ transplantation, diseases such as AIDS which predispose to opportunistic infections, and a greater frequency of invasive procedures of the biliary tract. Other groups at increased risk include diabetics, alcoholics, those with other gastrointestinal bacterial diseases (appendicitis, diverticulitis, infectious colitis), and the ever-increasing elderly population. Hematogenous seeding of infectious agents overwhelm the phagocytic capability of Küpffer's cells and give rise to abscess formation.

Etiopathogenesis: The most common route for development of hepatic abscess is metastatic spread to the liver through the portal venous system (46%) from a source in the splanchnic system. Cholangitis, especially when associated with endoscopic instrumentation, biliary stones, neoplasms, or biliary stenosis, serves as the primary focus of infection leading to the formation of liver abscesses (38–50%). Finally, the source of infection remains unknown in a subset of patients with "cryptogenic" hepatic abscess in whom a hematogenous pathogenesis is suspected either via the hepatic arterial inflow or portal venous inflow.

Hepatic abscesses may be single or multiple (Figs. 4.1 and 4.2) and thereby provide some clues to the etiopathogenesis. In nearly 70% of patients, involvement of the right lobe is attributed to the preferential flow of the mesenteric and portal venous flow. Involvement of the left lobe is associated more frequently with intra-hepatic stones (Fig. 4.3).

Besides its association with diseases described traditionally, such as diabetes, cirrhosis, biliary stones, colonic diverticulitis, and appendicitis, pyogenic liver abscesses are also associated with other medical conditions of more recent development. Abscess formation secondary to radio-frequency ablation of malignant primary or metastatic neoplasms ranges between 1% and 6%.

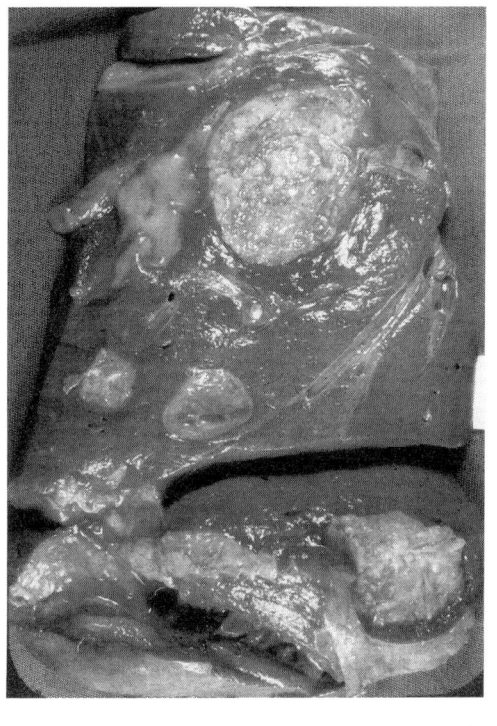

FIGURE 4.1. Pyogenic liver abscesses. Pathologic specimen. Note multiple focus.

A recent study of 603 patients with hepatocellular carcinoma treated with radio-frequency identified the risk factors associated with abscess formation to be pre-existing biliary abnormalities favoring ascending cholangitis, retention within the tumor of the ionized oil from the trans-arterial chemo-embolization, and prior cryotherapy treatment. In itself, transarterial embolization of malignant liver neoplasias has a very low rate (<0.5%) of liver abscess formation, but when it occurs, the organisms are usually gram-positive bacterial infections; others have suggested that patients with bacteriobilia related to previous instrumentation or bilioenteric anastomosis are also at increased risk.

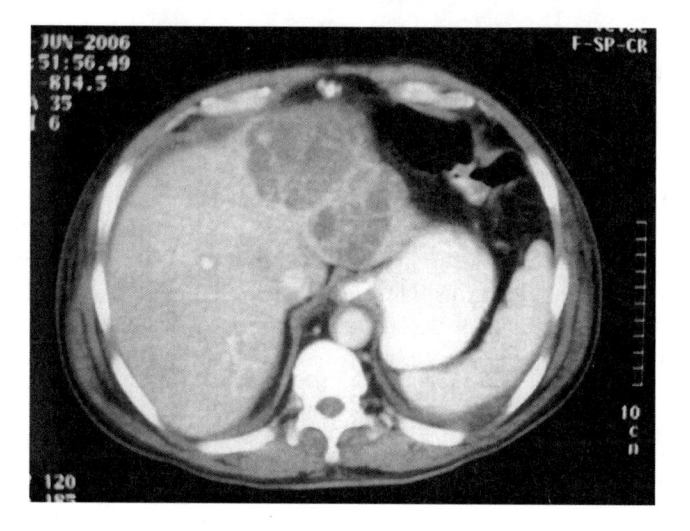

FIGURE 4.2. CT of pyogenic liver abscess. Note multiloculated abscess in segment II-III.

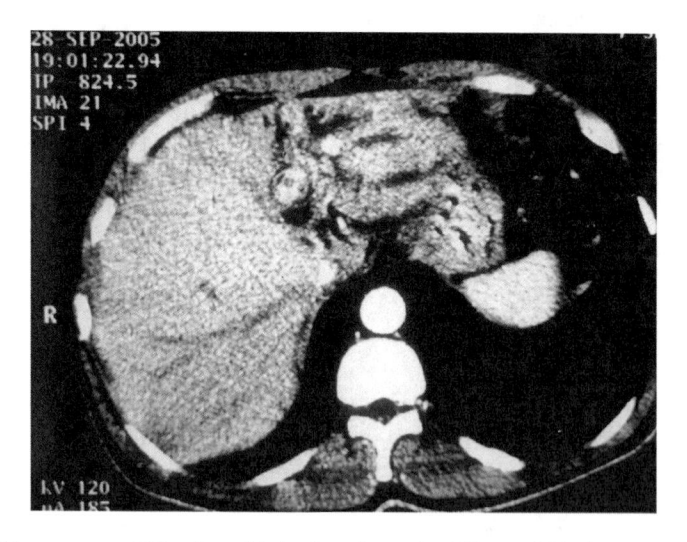

FIGURE 4.3. CT of multiple intrahepatic biliary lithiasis of left hepatic duct. Note presence of pyogenic liver microabscesses and atrophy.

The immunosuppressed populations are most at risk of developing liver abscess. Hematologic malignancies predispose to the development of metastatic infectious processes such as splenic abscess, brain abscess, and hepatic abscess, and especially fungal abscesses, both before and during treatment. Similarly, approximately 1% of patients with HIV infection will develop some form of hepatic abscess; the susceptibility appears to vary with the degree of immune compromise. In liver transplant patients, cytomegalovirus (CMV) infection of the liver is characterized by the formation of diffuse parenchymal abscesses usually containing Küpffer cells infected with the virus. In addition, the presence of CMV infection associated with immunosuppression also favors the presence of invasive aspergillosis. When the CD4 count is >500, the organisms involved are generally gram-negative aerobes, mainly Klebsiella species, followed by *E. coli* and Pseudomonas; when the CD4 count is <200, abscesses have a mixed flora or are secondary to microbes such as Mycobacterium, Nocardia, Aspergillus, and other opportunistic species.

The post-transplantation population represents a somewhat unique group; not only are they immunosuppressed, but the liver graft has suffered an element of ischemic insult, and the biliary tree has been instrumented or become colonized with bacteria secondary to a bilio-enteric anastomosis. Transplant patients, particularly liver transplant patients, may develop liver abscesses (approximately 1–4%). Two factors have been associated with the predisposition to abscess formation: hepatic artery thrombosis (66%) and the use of biliary drainage catheters or biliary instrumentation resulting in bacteriobilia or especially cholangitis.

Finally, the etiology of cryptogenic abscesses that occur in 10–20% of patients with hepatic abscesses has not been established clearly. Some groups have suggested that these types of hepatic abscesses arise from small infarctions or areas of thromboembolism that become superinfected by microbes derived from bacteremias of the portal system, or possibly from defects in the reticuloendothelial system where

there is a loss of the ability to clear opsonized particles from the circulation. Ultimately, abscess development depends on the interaction between the patient's immune system, the route of dissemination, and the virulence of the pathogen (Table 4.1).

Mortality: Despite the fact that patients with pyogenic liver abscesses have highly debilitating diseases, advances in early diagnosis, less invasive treatments, and more

TABLE 4.1. Pathogenesis of pyogenic liver abscesses.

Dissemination route	Etiology	Causing microbe
Hepatic artery	Bacteremic infection	Gram (+) aerobes
		Gram (−) aerobes
Portal vein	Benign or malignant gastrointestinal disease	Gram (−) aerobes Gram (−) anaerobes
Biliary tract	Cholangitis (stones, stent tumors, post-ERCP)	Gram (−) aerobes Gram (−) anaerobes
Round ligament	Umbilical piercing, umbilical catheter	Gram (+) aerobes
Liver parenchyma	Trauma, post radiofrequency	Gram (−) aerobes
Liver parenchyma	Transplant – arterial thrombosis	Gram (−) aerobes
		Cytomegalovirus
		Opportunistic germ
Mixed	AIDS, transplant, chemotherapy	Opportunistic germ
		Fungi
		Gram (−) aerobes
Continuity	Post-cholecystectomy, infection or perforation of neighboring organ	Gram (−) aerobes
		Gram (−) anaerobes
Cryptogenic	Unknown Dental diseases?	Gram (+) aerobes
		Gram (−) aerobes

sophisticated antimicrobial and supportive therapies have resulted in an overall decrease in mortality. Nevertheless, the following risk factors have been associated with increased hospital mortality: presence of malignancy, hyperbilirubinemia, increased partial thromboplastin time, hypoalbuminemia <2.5 g/dl, leukocytosis (>20,000 cells/mm³), and diabetes. One factor that increases mortality markedly is spontaneous abscess perforation which, though uncommon, occurs in approximately 5% of patients and is associated with abscess size >7.8 cm in diameter (P = 0.043), presence of intra-luminal gas (P <0.001), and involvement of the left lobe (P = 0.018).

Clinical presentation: Overall, the male-to-female ratio for pyogenic liver abscesses has a slight predominance in males. Clinical signs and symptoms of pyogenic liver abscesses are usually nonspecific and are related to the local and systemic response to the primary site of infection. Major symptoms include fever (80–100%) and abdominal pain, especially in the right upper quadrant (60–85%). Less common are nausea, vomiting, and weight loss. Physical findings vary widely and include right upper quadrant tenderness (50%), hepatomegaly (40%), and jaundice (30%). The presence of a pleural or pericardial effusion, ascites, or severe shock may be the initial manifestation of a severe complication of the liver abscess.

Liver abscesses caused by Klebsiella can be associated with endogenous endophthalmitis which, although uncommon, can progress rapidly to visual loss in spite of medical intervention. The main risk factor associated with this finding is a history of diabetes. Every patient with a liver abscess who complains of any ocular pain or visual disorders must be referred to the ophthalmologist immediately.

Standard laboratory tests reflect a generalized state of systemic infection. Leukocytosis is present in 60–70% of patients and is a poor prognostic factor when greater than 20,000 cells/mm³. Other findings may include hypoalbuminemia, anemia, and abnormal liver function tests depending on the duration of the disease prior to diagnosis. Abscess cultures

are positive in >70% of cases of which at least 50% are polymicrobial. Blood cultures are positive in 40% of cases.

Treatment: Treatment of pyogenic liver abscesses involves the following therapeutic modalities: (1) parenteral antibiotic therapy, (2) percutaneous drainage, (3) operative drainage, and/or (4) hepatic resection. Antibiotic therapy is the only constant treatment once the diagnosis is made, while selection of the other forms of treatment depends on the specific conditions of the patient.

One adverse prognostic factor associated with mortality is delay in starting antibiotic therapy. For that reason, once the diagnosis of a liver abscess is made, empiric treatment with parenteral, broad-spectrum antibiotics should be initiated until culture of the luminal content confirms the organism(s) involved, after which the antibiotic therapy can be focused on the organism(s) involved. Unlike amoebic liver abscesses that usually resolve with anti-amoebic treatment alone, pyogenic abscesses treated only with antibiotic therapy have an unacceptable mortality (20%). Some selected groups of patients may benefit from this single modality of therapy, usually involving patients with small single or multiple abscesses of biliary origin, children, CMV microabscesses, and those with a rapid clinical response to monotherapy without evidence of systemic infection. There is no exact duration of suggested antibiotic therapy in these select patients, and the decision to discontinue treatment is based on clinical improvement, absence of fever or leukocytosis, and resolution of the abscess on follow-up imaging studies.

The current gold standard for the management of pyogenic liver abscesses not amenable to treatment with antibiotic therapy alone is percutaneous aspiration with placement of a drainage catheter under image guidance. The best candidates are patients with single, well-defined abscesses <7 cm in diameter with no associated complications (bleeding, perforation) or signs of severe septicemia. In some patients, aspiration alone, in conjunction with effective antibiotic therapy, can prove successful; in one study of 115 patients with pyogenic liver abscess (averaging 7 cm in size) treated with antibiotic

therapy and percutaneous needle aspiration alone, the treatment was successful in 98%, with an average of two aspirations per patient, and in half the one aspiration was enough to achieve abscess control.

If symptoms persist for 2 or 3 days after percutaneous treatment or if the overall status of the patient worsens without any changes in the imaging studies, operative drainage should be considered. Factors associated with failure of percutaneous drainage include multiple or multiloculated abscesses, size greater than 7 cm, viscous fluid or substantial necrotic material, intracystic bleeding, and perforation of the abscess. Liver abscesses associated with choledocholithiasis or biliary sepsis initially are managed currently with percutaneous catheter drainage, although on occasions there is a need for sphincterotomy, stenting, or nasobiliary tube placement. Although some groups have reported irrigation of the abscess cavity with antibiotics, this form of treatment is neither widely accepted nor usually needed.

Operative treatment is reserved currently for patients who do not respond to antibiotic therapy and percutaneous drainage or in patients with complications secondary to catheter placement (abscess rupture, intracystic bleeding, peritonitis). The selection of either a laparoscopic approach or an open technique depends on the experience of the surgical team and the specific situation. Hepatectomy or left lobectomy may be the first modality of treatment in patients of liver abscesses secondary to recurrent intrahepatic biliary lithiasis.

Amoebic Abscess

Pathogenesis: Colonic amoebiasis occurs worldwide, but developing countries have been identified as endemic areas, especially those located in tropical and subtropical regions. Amoebic infestation is associated usually with malnutrition and poor sanitary conditions. Nevertheless, with globalization of the population, symptomatic infections are found in practically all parts of the world. Approximately 10% of the world

population is infected with some type of amoebas. In those countries where the incidence is high (Mexico, Brazil, Vietnam, Colombia), the rate of symptomatic infections ranges between 2% and 49%, of which only about 10% of colonized subjects develop some form of invasive amoebiasis. The primary extra-colonic manifestation of amoebiasis is liver abscess; interestingly, a recent history of colonic dysentery is rare; indeed, the hepatic abscess may occur several years after the primary infection or even without any clinical history of colitis.

The cystic form of the parasite is in a vegetative state, and once swallowed, it remains in the colon and develops into its trophozoite form. This form can invade the colonic mucosa, giving rise to the typical flash-shaped ulcers. From there, the trophozoite form of the parasite can reach the liver via portal circulation, resist complement lysis along the way, and colonize and infect the liver parenchyma; abscesses form through the action of proteolytic enzymes that destroy the parenchyma, creating thrombosis and microabscesses that grow in size. Although grossly purulent, the luminal content usually remains sterile, except in about 20% of patients in whom bacterial superinfection may occur.

Mortality: Mortality in patients with amoebic abscesses depends on the virulence of the parasite, the host's immune status, and, especially, the presence of complications. In non-complicated cases, mortality is <5% but increases markedly to 11–40% when there are complications.

In a series of 503 patients from China with amoebic liver abscesses, 110 (22%) perforated, including 79 that perforated into the pleuropulmonary space, 15 into the subphrenic space, 11 into the peritoneal cavity, and 5 into other anatomic areas such as the pericardium, abdominal wall, and chest wall. Some 45% of patients with perforations into the abdominal cavity died compared with 14% of those who had perforations into a different anatomic site. Most abscesses in the pleuropulmonary and subphrenic spaces were managed satisfactorily with metronidazole and percutaneous drainage. Of 501 amoebic abscesses reported from Mexico with chest complications, 326 ruptured through the diaphragm. Treatment was with

metronidazole plus emetine and drainage. Mortality in this group was 12%. In contrast, free perforation into the abdominal cavity is a strong predictor of mortality. Other predictors of poor prognosis include perforation into the pericardium, multiple abscesses, volume greater than 500 ml, encephalopathy, albumin < 2/dl, diabetes mellitus, and severe anemia.

Clinical Presentation: Amoebic liver abscesses are 10 times more common in males than in females and are found only rarely in children. Amoebic abscesses tend to occur in young individuals, and their incidence is greater during the summer months in endemic areas.

About 75% of amoebic abscesses present as a solitary lesion localized usually in the right lobe; however, in one series from India, the involvement was of the left lobe in a greater percentage of patients (Fig. 4.4). Unlike pyogenic abscesses, amoebic abscesses are more subacute, and it may take weeks for symptoms to appear. At first, symptoms are non-specific and usually include fever (remitting or intermittent but generally not generally than 40°C unless there is bacterial superinfection) and

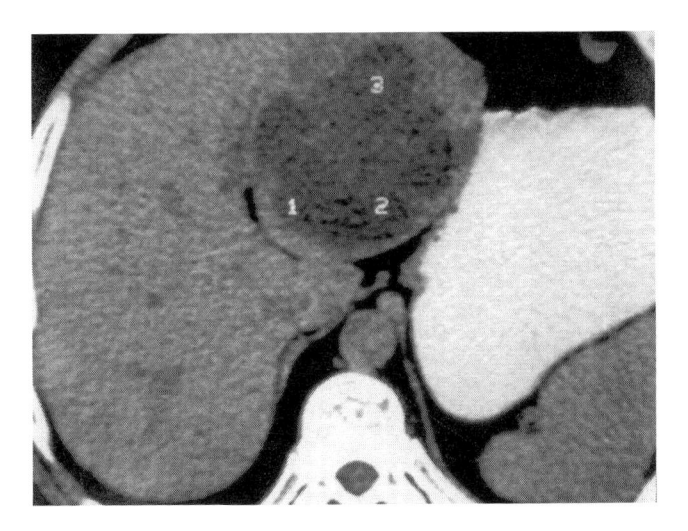

FIGURE 4.4. CT of amebic liver abscess. Note single abscess in segment II-III.

localized epigastric abdominal and right upper quadrant pain. When the abscess lies adjacent to the diaphragm, there may be referred shoulder pain, cough, or even pleurisy; right pleural effusion is present in 25–50% of cases. Deep abscesses may present with only fever and no other associated signs or symptoms. Gastrointestinal symptoms may be present in about 25% of patients and include nausea, vomiting, abdominal distension, and diarrhea, but concomitant colitis is rare.

More than 50% of patients have anemia as a function of a chronic process and an increased sedimentation rate. Moderate leukocytosis and neutrophilia are present in about 70% of patients. Liver function tests may be normal, but serum alkaline phosphatase and transaminase values may be increased slightly. Blood cultures, as well as cultures of the purulent, anchovy past-like intracystic material, are negative.

Indications, sensitivity, and specificity of the imaging studies are no different from those with pyogenic liver abscesses. Serum antibodies are of high, reliable diagnostic value for amoebic liver abscesses and are positive in 75% of patients in the acute phase and in >90% during the later phase. These tests remain positive for several months or even years afterward. Recent techniques of molecular biology directed at the serum, such as co-agglutination, ELISA, or polymerase chain reaction, may differentiate between recent and past infections, with reported sensitivities and specificities >90%. The co-agglutination test (Co-A) is a quick and easy way to determine the presence of circulating antigens in the serum of patients with amoebic liver abscess in 90% of cases, although there are problems with false positive results in patients with other parasitic or bacterial infections.

Treatment: The initial treatment of amoebic liver abscess involves a primary non-operative approach with antibiotics from the imidazole group, in particular metronidazole. The success rate with monotherapy ranges between 40% and 90%. Empiric response to the treatment with metronidazole also enables confirmation of the diagnosis of amebic liver abscess. There should be a rapid improvement of clinical symptoms, while radiologic changes become apparent only

7–10 days after the initiation of treatment. The radiologic signs of abscess and liver involvement disappear within 10–300 days, depending on the size and characteristics of the abscess. When there is no response to treatment with met-ronidazole, another possibility is to add chloroquine (600 mg/day for 2 days, followed by 300 mg/day for another 3 weeks) with or without paromomycin or diloxanide furoate. Dehydroemetine is considered the last line of treatment because of its high cardiac and gastrointestinal morbidity.

Percutaneous drainage with or without a catheter is per-formed only in patients who do not show any improvement with medical management and in other situations such as impending rupture, large left-lobe abscesses (>5–7 cm), suspi-cion of a bacterial superinfection, and ultrasonographic con-firmation of a largely fluid collection. The success of the combined therapy is >90%; laparoscopic or open drainage is reserved for otherwise untreatable complications.

Considering that there is no animal reservoir or vector for Entamoeba histolytica, theoretically a vaccine could poten-tially eliminate intestinal infections and, consequently, amoe-bic liver abscesses. Immunologic assessments have shown that specific protection against amoebic infections is associated with the production of antibodies against the adhesion mol-ecule lectin, an antigenic protein found in 95% of the infec-tious strains of Entamoeba histolytica. Experimental studies in animal models using immunologic therapies directed at galactose and N-acetyl-D-galactosamine, lectin, serine-rich proteins, cysteine proteases, lipophosphoglycanes, amoe-bapores, and protein 29-kDA have proven to be effective immunoprotection, thus constituting the future prophylactic treatments for Entamoeba histolytica infections, a disease that could be prevented by improving sanitation designed to avoid fecal contamination of water and food sources.

Selected Readings

Choi D, Lim HK, Kim MJ, et al. (2005) Liver abscess after percutaneous radiofrequency ablation for hepatocellular carcinoma: frequency and risk factors. AJR Am J Roentgenol 184:1860–1867

Chu KM, Fan ST, Lai EC, et al. (1996) Pyogenic liver abscess. An audit of experience over the past decade. Arch Surg 131:148–152

Haque R, Huston CD, Hughes M, et al. (2003) Current concepts: amebiasis. New Engl J Med 348:1565–1573

Huang CJ, Pitt HA, Lipsett PA, et al. (1996) Pyogenic hepatic abscess. Changing trends over 42 years. Ann Surg 223:600–607; discussion 607–609

Hughes MA, Petri WA Jr. (2000) Amebic liver abscess. Infect Dis Clin North Am 14:546–582

Kim W, Clark TW, Baum RA, Soulen MC (2001) Risk factors for liver abscess formation after hepatic chemoem-bolization. J Vasc Interv Radiol 12:965–968

Rahimian J, Wilson T, Oram V, Holzman RS (2004) Pyogenic liver abscess: recent trends in etiology and mortality. Clin Infect Dis 39:21654–1659

5
Portal Hypertension

Héctor Orozco and Miguel Angel Mercado

Pearls and Pitfalls

- Portal hypertension has various etiologies, each with a particular pathophysiology that may impact treatment options.
- Extrahepatic portal hypertension is secondary to portal thrombosis and is associated frequently with disorders of coagulation (protein C, protein S, or antithrombin III deficiencies).
- In hepatic cirrhosis, the obstructive process is intrahepatic, leading to increases in both vascular resistance and splanchnic vasodilatation.
- There is no specific prophylaxis that will prevent portal hypertension-induced variceal formation; however, for primary prophylaxis (to try to prevent variceal bleeding), the treatment of choice is β-blockade, although endoscopic treatment of varices may be considered.
- For secondary prophylaxis (recurrent bleeding), the first line treatments are β-blockade and endoscopic procedures with band ligation.
- Transjugular Intrahepatic Portosystemic Shunt (TIPS) is a second line procedure used in refractory patients after failed endoscopic therapy and as a bridge to hepatic transplantation.

K.I. Bland et al. (eds.), *Liver and Biliary Surgery*,
DOI 10.1007/978-1-84996-429-6_5,
© Springer-Verlag London Limited 2011

- Surgical intervention may be recommended as a secondary prophylaxis in patients with early failure of medical management and good hepatic function (Child-Pugh A-B).
- Operative procedures that preserve prograde portal (hepatopedal) flow are the procedures of choice.
- Non-selective shunts are effective for control of hemorrhage, but the incidence of encephalopathy is high.
- In our experience, the distal splenorenal shunt is the preferred surgical option with reservation of extensive devascularization procedures for situations of inappropriate anatomy (splenic thrombosis).
- Liver transplantation is reserved for patients with refractory bleeding and poor liver function (Child-Pugh C).

Introduction

Increased pressure in the portal venous system is known as portal hypertension (PH). Normal total hepatic blood flow is about 2 l/min but comes from two sources; the hepatic artery contributes about 600–700 ml/min and the portal venous system about 1,300 ml/minute. The portal venous system supplies 75% of the oxygen delivery to the liver with the remainder from the hepatic artery.

PH is a combination of increased resistance at the hepatic sinusoidal level and an increase in total hepatic blood flow. The production of vasoactive substances at the hepatic sinusoids also contributes to these hemodynamic changes. In the setting of PH, there is also an increased pressure within the lymphatic system that can contribute to the development of ascites as well. The main consequences of PH are bleeding from gastro-esophageal varices and hypersplenism (leukopenia, anemia, and thrombocytopenia).

The most common conditions leading to PH in adults are alcohol abuse, viral infection-induced cirrhosis, and venous thrombosis, while in Africa, the Middle East, and South America, hepatic fibrosis due to schistosomiasis is equally common.

Etiopathogenesis

Intrahepatic PH: In most Western countries, the cirrhosis leading to intrahepatic PH is related either to alcohol abuse or viral hepatitis (usually hepatitis B or C) leading to cirrhosis. With increasing frequency, however, non-alcoholic steato-hepatitis (NASH) is becoming a more common etiology of advanced cirrhosis (accounting for as much as 20% of all cirrhotics in the United States), probably related to the increased prevalence of obesity worldwide. Other more unusual etiologies include hemochromatosis, α-1 anti-trypsin deficiency, Wilson's disease, etc.

Extrahepatic PH: PH can occur from obstruction or thrombosis of venous inflow to or from the liver. The main causes of posthepatic, extrahepatic PH are obstruction of the hepatic veins, inferior vena cava, or both, as in the Budd-Chiari syndrome (hepatic outflow occlusive disease).

Prehepatic extrahepatic PH is due primarily to thrombosis of the portal vein. This disorder can occur in children with omphalitis; however, many of these children have idiopathic portal hypertension. Not infrequently, these patients will also have histologic and functional hepatic abnormalities even though the macroscopic features of the liver appear to be normal. It is possible that these children have idiopathic PH and that the portal thrombosis is only one of the stages of the disease.

Another cause of extrahepatic PH is thrombosis of the splenic vein, which leads to a segmental increase in extrahepatic venous pressure termed sinistral, or "left-sided" PH. This segmental PH occurs most frequently as a complication of pancreatitis, although other causes include pancreatic neoplasms or trauma. This segmental increase in venous outflow of the spleen leads to intrasplenic venous hypertension, which induces the development of venous collaterals of drainage through the stomach via the short gastric veins leading to gastric varices. Rare causes of prehepatic PH include iatrogenic or spontaneous arterio-portal fistulae that may occur after percutaneous hepatic biopsies, percutaneous biliary intubation, or secondary

to visceral aneurysms. Finally, primary thrombosis may occur in the setting of thrombophilias such as deficiencies in Protein C, Protein S, and anti-thrombin III autoimmune pathologies (antiphospholid antibodies), and other hematologic abnormalities such as paroxysmal nocturnal hemoglobinuria. These abnormalities can cause both pre-and posthepatic PH.

For many years, the belief was that rupture of esophageal varices was the only cause of bleeding. Nowadays, we know that bleeding from gastric varices is also a frequent cause. In these patients, it is common to find a congestive gastropathy as well.

The portal pressure should be considered dynamic rather than static, because abrupt increases in pressure in the portal system are frequent. These increases are transmitted to the varicose plexus by everyday life activities such as sneezing, physical exertion, or defecation. Hemodynamic studies with a catheter in the portal vein demonstrate that the Valsalva maneuver can increase the portal pressure by 20–60 mm of pressure.

Clinical Manifestations

The main signs and symptoms suggestive of PH are abdominal collateral circulation, evidence of esophageal varices, abdominal ascites, and splenomegaly. In more recent times, endoscopic ultrasonography has been used to classify varices and identify collateral circulation. CT and Doppler ultrasonography may better define the areas of the hepatic or splenic helium; these two diagnostic methods have the advantage of being non-invasive.

The most severe consequence of PH is esophageal hemorrhage from the thin-walled esophageal varices. Nevertheless, not all patients with PH experience esophageal bleeding. Only 15–30% of all the patients with cirrhosis, PH, and esophagogastric varices will develop variceal hemorrhage.

Diagnosis

After a thorough clinical and physical examination, determination of underlying liver disease and defining the etiology for the PH (pre-, intra-or posthepatic) is imperative. Laboratory

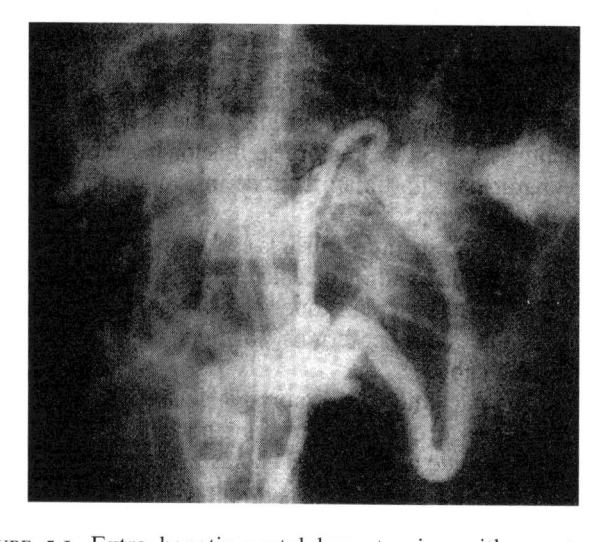

FIGURE 5.1. Extra hepatic portal hypertension with spontaneous spleno-renal shunt.

evaluation, radiologic imaging, and endoscopic means are the most fruitful. Angiographic studies, although invasive, are necessary occasionally for rare causes of PH (Fig. 5.1). The goals are to define the presence/absence of hepatic parenchymal disease (e.g. cirrhosis; see Chapter 1), the site of portal venous obstruction (intrahepatic, hepatic venous outflow, extrahepatic portal system, etc.), and the presence or absence of esophageal, gastric, and/or small bowel varices.

Treatment

Surgical treatment of PH is usually indicated only in patients who have failed medical management, with the goal of avoiding recurrent bleeding. Operative intervention as prophylaxis in select, high-risk patients without prior complications has been advocated by some authors but remains highly controversial, and most studies of prophylactic operative decompression have not shown an advantage in overall survival. In contrast, prophylactic treatment for the patient with PH is based in the use of

drugs such as β-blockers or those that modify the cardiac output, systemic blood pressure, and portal pressure. Several prospective studies have demonstrated the ability of β-blockers to reduce variceal bleeding complications compared with placebo. Currently, there are prospective studies suggesting the value of prophylactic endoscopic banding of the varicose plexus in patients without prior variceal hemorrhage; variceal banding is useful in patients with contraindications to or intolerance of pharmacologic prophylactic measures.

Treatment of PH is based on presence or absence of symptoms, etiology, extent of liver disease, and prior treatments. If varices are present, specific treatment should be considered, including pharmacologic therapy, sclerotherapy, or transjugular intrahepatic shunting (TIPS). Under conditions of active variceal hemorrhage, the options include emergency sclerotherapy, balloon tamponade, emergency TIPS, or surgical therapy (portosystemic shunts, devascularization procedures, or even hepatic transplantation).

Pharmacologic treatment: Several studies have demonstrated that vasopressin decreases the pressure of the portal system and produces constriction of the muscular esophageal walls with collapse of the gastroesophageal varices. Given the short half-life of vasopressin, continuous IV infusions are required.

The combination of nitroglycerin and vasopressin may help to control not only the portal hypertension but also will protect the patient with coronary artery disease from the cardiac side-effects of a vasoconstrictive agent. This treatment may have some adverse effects, such as lowering the blood pressure that may lead to other complications. Other drugs such as somatostatin or its homologues are relatively effective for the control of acute bleeding and appear equally effective as sclerotherapy and/or variceal banding in prospective controlled trials.

Balloon tamponade: A useful maneuver for controlling acute, severe bleeding from esophageal varices is to place a transoral balloon tamponade system such as the Blakemore-Sengstaken tube or the Minnesota tube. These tubes have an external balloon that applies pressure directly on the varices

when the balloon is inflated in the gastric and/or esophageal lumen. Balloon tamponade is used only in the emergency situation when the bleeding cannot be controlled by other measures. Use of these tubes is limited and requires intensive care unit monitoring. With some of the newer techniques discussed below, balloon tamponade is used only rarely today.

Sclerotherapy and variceal banding: Endoscopic sclerotherapy and banding are effective in controlling acute variceal bleeding in up to 95% of patients. In addition, they also allow stabilization of patients who may require a more definitive procedure. Because recurrent variceal bleeding occurs in up to 40% of patients after sclerotherapy or variceal banding, the addition of pharmacologic treatment decrease recurrence of bleeding.

Transjugular intrahepatic shunt (TIPS): Placement of an intrahepatic shunt creating a fistula between a branch of the portal vein with a hepatic vein is accomplished through transjugular transhepatic venous approach and is known as a TIPS procedure. This procedure is carried out percutaneously under fluoroscopic control. The catheter is positioned retrograde into a hepatic vein; from this position and through this catheter, a needle is advanced through the hepatic parenchyma until an intrahepatic portal vein with adequate caliber is accessed. After that, this track is dilated, and an 8–10 cm circular metallic endoprosthesis is placed. This prosthesis/shunt allows decompression of the PH through the shunt into the low pressure vena cava.

Theoretically, TIPS is an ideal treatment option for decompressing the portal system in patients with poor liver function, abnormalities in coagulation, ascites, jaundice, and even encephalopathy, where operative risks would be substantial. Potential advantages of TIPS are that it avoids the need for an operative portosystemic shunt in the very high risk patients and does not alter surgical anatomy in candidates for a liver transplantation. Potential disadvantages of TIPS include the need for specialists in interventional radiology and the risks of encephalopathy or liver failure. Indeed, development of encephalopathy after TIPS may accelerate the need for liver

transplantation. Other risks include the possibility of hepatic vein or portal vein thrombosis, which may lead to obstacles for future liver transplantation, or shunt occlusion which occurs in up to 30% of patients within the first year after placement. The use of "protected" or "coated" stents appears to decrease the incidence of stent occlusion.

Emergency surgical treatment: Operative intervention in patients who arrive in the emergency room with severe bleeding secondary to hepatic cirrhosis is associated with a very high mortality rate. Procedural options include portosystemic shunts (selective and non-selective) and devascularization procedures. Non-selective shunts offer excellent control of PH and ascites but have an increased risk of inducing or worsening encephalopathy. These procedures include end-to-end or side-to-side portocaval shunts or the mesocaval shunt.

Devascularization procedures have been advocated by some for the emergent treatment of patients with bleeding. These procedures involve transmural or direct ligation of esophageal varices, transaction and reanastomosis of the esophagus to disrupt continuity of gastroesophageal varices, esophagogastric resections, and esophagogastric devascularization. While these procedures have some merit in the emergent management of patients with bleeding esophageal varices, the long-term outcome is much less favorable; surviving patients exhibit a high incidence of recurrent bleeding. In the emergent setting, operative intervention in patients with Childs C cirrhosis is contraindicated. These patients are best treated with nonsurgical methods described previously, including TIPS. On occasion, patients with prehepatic PH from schistosomiasis or portal venous thrombosis may benefit in the acute setting from an esophagogastric devascularization procedure such as the Sugiura-Futagawa operation.

In an elective setting in patients with preserved liver function and a patent, anatomically appropriate portal anatomy, the treatment of choice is total porto-systemic shunt via portacaval shunt (end-side or side-side), a side-to-side splenorenal shunt, or a mesocaval shunt. One operative procedure

that may stop variceal bleeding is the small diameter mesocaval or portocaval "H" shunt with a small diameter graft. According to Sarfeh and colleagues, this type of "semi-selective" shunt is capable of partial decompression of the portal system without complete diversion of the hepatic portal flow. Probably the most attractive portal decompressive procedure is the distal splenorenal shunt, also called the Warren shunt. The "selective" distal splenorenal shunt is technically more demanding and time-consuming and is used rarely in the emergent setting.

Devascularization procedures, such as described by Sugiura and Futagawa, are successful in the management of acute variceal bleeding and have the advantages of a decrease in operative mortality, avoidance of encephalopathy induced by shunts, and do not require preoperative vascular imaging. In an elective setting, these procedures are best used in patients with schistosomiasis and not cirrhosis.

Selection of Patients for Elective Operative Management

The clinical evaluation of patients considered for operative intervention to correct complications of PH is critical. It is imperative to determine the underlying liver function, Childs class, MELD score, and other potential prohibitive comorbidities in all patients. Evaluation includes laboratory, endoscopic, and imaging tests.

Laboratory studies include the concentrations of serum glucose, urea, creatinine, and electrolytes, hematologic studies, complete liver function tests, coagulation parameters (prothrombin time), and platelet count. Endoscopic evaluation is also necessary to evaluate the presence of esophageal or gastric varices, congestive gastropathy, and any other gastric or duodenal abnormalities. Radiologic evaluation may include ultrasonography to assess liver parenchyma, hepatic vasculature, and direction of portal venous flow.

Once this preliminary evaluation has been completed, the next step is to decide which operative procedure is best suited

to the patient. To facilitate this decision, angiographic studies are recommended that together are called hepatic panangiography. In the past, angiography included a celiac artery injection along with the venous phase to determine the patency and anatomy of the portal venous system; when appropriate, the vena cava and left renal vein was also imaged to determine its distance from the splenic vein. Currently, CT angiography and magnetic resonance angiography are often able to define satisfactorily the vascular anatomy without the invasiveness of angiography.

Hepatic venography can serve as an indirect evaluation of the hepato-portal flow; at the same time it is allows assessment of pressure gradients between the portal and systemic systems. The pressure measurements made are the wedge hepatic pressure, which estimates closely the portal vein pressure; the "corrected portal pressure" or transhepatic pressure gradient can then be calculated using the difference between the wedge pressure and the pressure in the inferior vena caval; normal "corrected" portal pressure is <5 mmHg.

In patients with chronic liver disease and PH with preservation of portal hepatic flow, a selective shunt is the preferred procedure. The "selective" shunts include the distal splenorenal or "Warren" shunt or alternatively an "H" type mesocaval shunt with a small diameter (8 mm) graft. In those patients with sinistral hypertension due to splenic vein thrombosis *without* liver disease, splenectomy is generally curative. When there is concomitant thrombosis of both splenic and superior mesenteric veins, the Sugiura procedure may be used, beginning with the abdominal approach, and 4–6 weeks later completed with the thoracic approach. A modification of the Sugiura-Futagawa procedure which we call "complete porto-azygous disconnection," involves an abdominal devascularization with subsequent endoscopic eradication of esophageal varices via banding.

Porto-systemic shunts: The non-selective porto-systemic shunts, such as the portocaval, central splenorenal, mesocaval with an "H" or "C" graft, and portorenal shunts decompress completely the portal system and control hemorrhage very

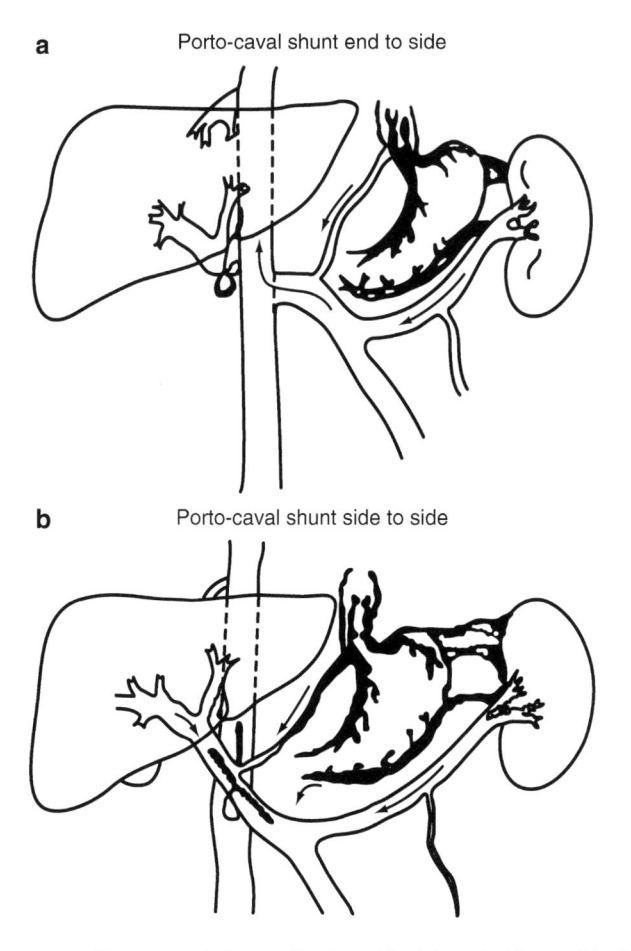

FIGURE 5.2. Porto-caval shunts. End to side (**a**) and side to side (**b**).

effectively. But as a result of the extent of diversion of portal flow, these total shunts are associated with an increased risk of encephalopathy, because they divert essentially all portal venous flow away from the liver (Fig. 5.2). To reduce this risk of encephalopathy, several authors have advocated the use of an intervening small diameter graft (<8 mm) to provide resistance to total diversion and to preserve at least some portal flow.

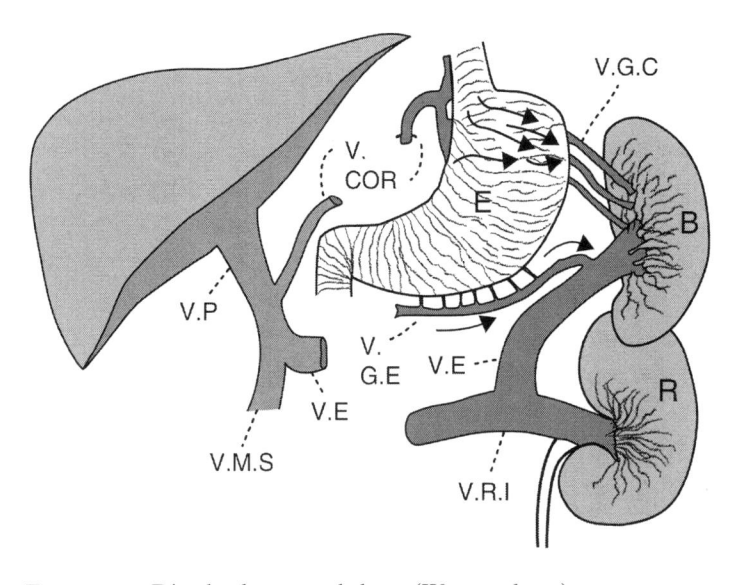

FIGURE 5.3. Distal spleno-renal shunt (Warren shunt).

With the conventional, non-selective porto-systemic shunts, the risk of hepatic encephalopathy in the postoperative period can reach 40–50% in patients with compromised hepatic function (Childs B and C). In contrast, the selective porto-systemic shunts, such as the distal splenorenal shunt or Warren shunt (Fig. 5.3) decompresses the varices in the esophagogastric area without altering hepatic portal flow from the superior mesenteric vein (and gut blood flow), at least acutely. With longer follow-up, many patients will develop venous collateral connections with the pancreatic veins in an attempt to decompress the "preserved" portal pressure, thereby partially reversing the selective nature of the operation.

Budd-Chiari Syndrome: In patients with hepatic venous outflow obstruction leading to posthepatic PH in whom the inferior vena cava is not affected, a conventional non-selective porto-systemic shunt, such as a side-to-side portocaval or mesocaval "H" or "C" graft, will decompress the PH effectively. In contrast, when the hepatic hypertrophy of the caudate lobe

causes compression of the inferior vena cava or when there is an inferior vena caval web or thrombosis, portocaval or meso-caval shunts are contraindicated, and alternatives such as a mesoatrial shunt with a graft must be considered. Some groups have shown that not every patient with Budd-Chiari syndrome requires operative intervention due to development of sponta-neous portosystemic shunts in some patients. Surgical treat-ment was reserved for those patients with evidence of hepatic tissue necrosis on biopsy, which portends a poor prognosis without operative intervention. Conversely, others suggest that hepatic necrosis will develop in most if not all patients with Budd-Chiari syndrome and recommend operative interven-tion to avoid eventual hepatic failure.

In the setting of acute, severe, hepatic necrosis, liver trans-plantation is necessary, however, due to the possibility of recurrent thrombosis, we recommend lifelong anticoagula-tion after transplantation for Budd-Chiari syndrome.

The most recent alternative to treat this problem is the placement of a TIPS. Endoluminal rechanneling of the hepatic vein with subsequent placement of a portoatrial expandable coated stent is another possibility.

Esophagogastric devascularization: When a porto-systemic shunt is contraindicated, esophagogastric devascularization (Sugiura-Futagawa) or complete porto-azygous disconnec-tion may be considered. In the authors' experience of more than 1,000 patients with mean follow-up of 10 years, esoph-agogastric devascularization can be performed with low rates of postoperative morbidity and mortality. The mortality rate of 25% in the emergency setting is considerable compared with 2% in the elective setting. Postoperative encephalopathy occurs in less than 5% of patients and recurrent bleeding in 10%. Estimated 3-year survival is 85%.

The Sugiura-Futagawa procedure consists of an extensive esophageal and gastric devascularization from the area of the left inferior pulmonary vein of the thoracic esophagus to the lesser curvature of the stomach; this devascularization is com-pleted with transaction of the lower third of the esophagus with reanastomosis, combined with splenectomy, pyloroplasty, and gastric devascularization. In general, this treatment

approach is done in two stages. In young people with adequate hepatic function and PH without cirrhosis, this procedure can be done in one stage.

The authors have utilized a modification of the Sugiura-Futagawa technique. Instead of dissecting and devascularizing just the lesser curvature, the gastro hepatic ligament, left gastric (coronary) vein and artery, and all the structures to the abdominal esophagus and fundus and body of the stomach are divided (Fig. 5.4). In addition, the right gastric vein and artery are ligated in three different places along the lesser curvature with non-absorbable sutures. The major curvature of the stomach is completely devascularized except for the right gastroepiploic artery; this devascularization is done with preservation of the spleen. For the thoracic stage, the esophageal transaction was modified. Instead of transecting the esophageal mucosa in its entire circumference, as described by Sugiura, we divide the anterior muscular layer, free the mucosa in its entire circumference, and perform a complete circular suture; in so doing, we ligate all the variceal plexus, diminishing the possibility of a postoperative esophageal fistula. The last modification is ligation of the right gastroepiploic vein distal to the pylorus. These modifications have been called a complete porto-azygous disconnection. Given the

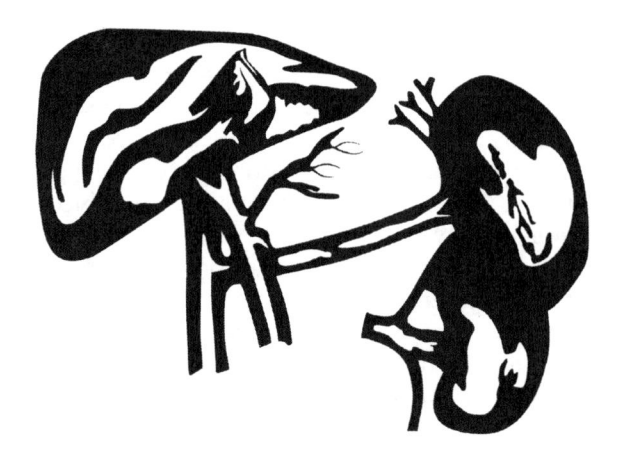

FIGURE 5.4. Complete porto-azygous disconnection.

effectiveness of endoscopic obliteration of the esophageal variceal plexus, we now perform the abdominal phase of the complete porto-azygous disconnection and then perform endoscopic variceal banding instead of the traditional second stage, transthoracic operation.

Prevention and Treatment of Hepatic Failure After Operation

One of the major concerns in the operative management of patients with PH is hepatic failure after operation. Careful patient selection and preoperative preparation is essential. During the operation, it is important that hemodynamic stability be maintained. The procedure must be performed with meticulous dissection to avoid hemorrhage resulting in hypovolemia and hypoxia which may exacerbate any potential hepatic injury. Crystalloid administration must be controlled carefully during the operation to avoid fluid retention and promote or worsen ascites in the postoperative period. Frequently, colloid solutions or albumin are used postoperatively to avoid excessive administration of crystalloid. Narcotics, sedatives, or hypnotics are used with reservation, and high protein consumption is avoided in the early postoperative period. In some instances, oral or rectal lactulose and non-absorbable oral antibiotics (neomycin) are required to avoid hepatic pre coma or ammonium intoxication. In general, in well-selected patients with preserved hepatic function undergoing elective surgery for PH, it is rare that additional treatments for hepatic insufficiency are necessary.

Hepatic transplantation: Hepatic transplantation offers potential definitive treatment of hepatic cirrhosis, PH, and resulting bleeding varices. Hepatic transplantation is not indicated in patients with adequate hepatic function when their only problem is bleeding, given the limited organ availability and the favorable results of shunts and devascularization procedures in these patients. Other factors that influence the decision for hepatic transplantation are the etiology of the hepatic disease, organ availability, presence of a small hepatocellular carcinoma, and psychosocial factors of patients with alcoholic liver disease.

Selected Readings

Abraldes JG, Angermayr B, Bosch J (2005) The management of portal hypertension. Clin Liver Dis 9:685–713

García-Tsao G (2006) Portal hypertension. Curr Opin Gas-troenterol 22:254–262

Henderson JM, Yang Y (2005) Is there still a role for surgery in bleeding portal hypertension? Nat Clin Pract Gastroenterol Hepatol 2(6):246–247

Klupp J, Kohler S, Pascher A, Neuhaus P (2005) Liver transplantation as ultimate tool to treat portal hypertension. Dig Dis 23:65–75

Mercado MA, Orozco H, Chan C, et al. (2004) Surgical treatment of non-cirrhotic presinusoidal portal hypertension. Hepatogastroenterology 51:1757–1760

Rosemurgy AX, Osborne D, Zervos EE (2005) Portal hypertension: the role of shunting procedures. Adv Surg 39:315–329

Vignali C, Bargellini I, Grosso M, et al. (2005) TIPS with expanded poly-tetracluoroethylene covered stent: results of an Italian multicenter study. Am J Roentgenol 185:472–480

6
Cystic Liver Diseases

Catherine Hubert, Laurence Annet, Bernard E.VanBeers, Yves Horsmans, and Jean-Franççois Gigot

Pearls and Pitfalls

- The most common cystic diseases of the liver are congenital liver cysts (CLCs), parasitic liver cysts, and cystic liver tumors.
- Appropriate diagnosis of the cyst is mandatory before treatment, since management options vary, ranging from observation to radical resection.
- Patient history, imaging studies, serological markers, and cyst-fluid analysis when a parasitic liver cyst has been excluded, are key factors for making an appropriate differential diagnosis of cystic liver disease.
- Uncertain diagnosis is often encountered between a complicated CLC and a neoplastic cyst.
- Liver cystadenoma is a rare but either overtly or potentially malignant lesion, requiring radical excision.
- A tailored surgical treatment is indicated for patients suffering from cystic liver lesions, ranging from fenestration to resection.
- Because the natural history of CLC is benign, treatment options should be discussed only when cysts are large in size or strategically located *and* when specific cyst-related symptoms or complications are present.

K.I. Bland et al. (eds.), *Liver and Biliary Surgery*,
DOI 10.1007/978-1-84996-429-6_6,
© Springer-Verlag London Limited 2011

- The causal relationship between abdominal pain and the presence of a large CLC should always be questioned before surgical treatment.
- When doubt persists concerning supposed cyst-related abdominal pain from a large CLC, percutaneous cyst aspiration should be performed as a pretherapeutic test. If abdominal complaints resolve after percutaneous aspiration (and recur with cyst recurrence), symptoms can be reasonably attributed to the cystic disease. Otherwise, another cause should be searched for.
- Missing the diagnosis of liver cystadenoma and thus adopting a conservative treatment leads to recurrence, sometimes as a malignant lesion.
- Macroscopic and microscopic examinations of the cyst wall with routine frozen section are key factors during surgery to differentiate between benign complicated congenital and neoplastic liver cysts.
- The diagnosis of neoplastic liver cyst is a formal indication for surgical treatment, even if the patient is free of symptoms.
- Precise ultrasonographic classification of hydatid liver cyst allows the choice of a tailored treatment strategy.

Introduction

Cystic lesions of the liver are commonly encountered in clinical practice as a result of the patient's accessibility to modern non-invasive imaging techniques. Cystic liver lesions can be broadly divided into four categories: congenital, traumatic, parasitic, and neoplastic (Table 6.1). Disease prevalence is broadly different for each type, with congenital liver cysts (CLCs) being the most frequent. The natural history and the risk of malignant transformation are completely different for the various types of cystic liver diseases. Appropriate diagnosis of hepatic cyst is thus essential to enable the physician to plan the correct treatment, which ranges from observation for asymptomatic CLCs to radical resection for cystic liver neoplasms. Differential diagnosis is based on the clinical history, imaging studies, and sometimes on sampling of intracystic fluid.

TABLE 6.1. Classification of cystic liver diseases.

- *Congenital liver cysts*
  - Simple
  - Polycystic disease
  - Biliary hamartoma (microhamartoma, von Meyenburg complex)
  - Ciliated hepatic foregut cyst
- *Parasitic liver cysts*
  - Echinococcal cyst (hydatid disease)
- *Neoplastic liver cysts*
  - Primary
    - Cystadenoma
    - Cystadenocarcinoma
    - Cystic mesenchymal hamartoma
  - Secondary
    - Cystic metastases from sarcoma, melanoma, lung, breast, mucinous colorectal, neuroendocrine tumors
    - Large necrosed primary tumors (hepatocellular carcinoma etc.)
- Acquired liver cysts
  - Posttraumatic hematoma or biloma
  - Liver abscess

Classification of Cystic Liver Diseases

Congenital Liver Cysts

CLCs are cystic formations, containing crystal-clear fluid when uncomplicated, with no communication to the intrahepatic bile ducts. CLCs are considered to develop from dilatation of aberrant intrahepatic bile ducts during embryogenesis. Microscopically, CLCs are lined by a single layer of cuboid or columnar epithelium, resembling biliary epithelial cells.

The small cysts are surrounded by normal hepatic tissue but large cysts can produce atrophy of the adjacent tissue. The disease is common with a prevalence of 1–5% in the general population, but is reported to be more frequent in women. The lesions may be solitary or multiple, vary from a few milli-meters to several centimeters in diameter, and are usually unilocular. Few lesions are really huge in size or potentially responsible for producing symptoms. The natural history of CLC is benign regarding disease progression. Most CLCs, even large lesions, are discovered incidentally in asymptom-atic patients and do not require any treatment.

Only 10–15% of large CLCs will become symptomatic or complicated. The most common symptoms are upper abdomi-nal discomfort and pain. However, the causal relationship between abdominal pain or discomfort and a benign CLC should always be questioned and accepted only if the cyst is large enough and after other possible causes of the symptoms have been excluded. In cases of doubt, a percutaneous aspira-tion test should be used to ensure that symptoms resolve with cyst aspiration. In most cases, liver function is entirely normal. Complications of large CLCs are uncommon but include com-pression of adjacent organs (biliary tract, stomach, or duode-num), intracystic hemorrhage or infection, posttraumatic rupture and torsion of pedunculated cysts. Hemorrhage is the most common complication, revealed by sudden acute abdom-inal pain with tense and painful hepatomegaly. However, the frequent finding of brownish intracystic fluid suggests that subclinical hemorrhage is probably more frequent than previ-ously thought. Spontaneous cyst infection is exceptional and is caused usually by repeated percutaneous drainage. The typical radiological appearances are modified in complicated CLCs, leading to difficulties in the differential diagnosis with cystic liver neoplasm. Indications for treating CLCs include highly and specifically symptomatic or complicated large cysts.

Polycystic Liver Disease

Adult polycystic liver disease (PLD) is a rare, inherited auto-somal recessive disease, and is characterized by the presence of

numerous cysts scattered throughout the liver parenchyma. However, liver failure is exceptional. It is generally accepted that hepatic cysts in patients with PLD result from cystic dilatation of biliary microhamartomas that originate from von Meyenburg's complexes. The disease prevalence in autopsy series is between 0.05% and 0.53%, with a female preponderance. The disease is usually associated with polycystic kidney disease (PKD) and coexistent cerebrovascular aneurysms are seen in up to 10–20% of the patients. The prognosis of PLD is usually related to end-stage renal insufficiency due to PKD and to the occurrence of cerebral hemorrhage. A routine search for intracranial aneurysms is thus advocated in PLD patients.

The clinical course of PLD is slowly progressive, with gradual increasing liver volume and compression of adjacent organs. Most PLD patients remain asymptomatic for a long period of time. When present, the commonest symptoms are related to gross polycystic hepatomegaly. These include chronic dull abdominal pain, abdominal discomfort, early satiety and supine dyspnea, leading to progressive physical disability in the individual's daily activities and professional life. Complications of PLD are uncommon, including acute intracystic hemorrhage and cyst infection, but are often severe with compressive complications such as biliary obstruction, portal hypertension, inferior vena caval compression, and hepatic venous outflow obstruction (Budd-Chiari syndrome).

Indications for surgery are restricted to selected patients with incapacitating or complicated polycystic hepatomegaly. The choice of surgical treatment is dictated by the cyst number, size, and distribution within the liver and by the complications of the disease. Our group reported a practical classification of PLD based on the number and size of the liver cysts and the amount of remaining normal liver parenchyma. Type I PLD includes patients with a limited number (<10) of large cysts (>10 cm), a situation that is quite similar to multiple CLCs with a huge dominant liver cyst. Type II PLD is represented by patients with diffuse involvement of the liver parenchyma by multiple medium-sized cysts with remaining large areas of noncystic liver parenchyma on preoperative CT. Type III PLD is a severe form of PLD with massive, diffuse involvement of

the liver parenchyma by small-and medium-sized liver cysts and only a few areas of preserved liver parenchyma between the cysts. To evaluate the results of surgical treatment, liver volumetry should be used from preoperative and serial post-operative abdominal CT.

Parasitic Hydatid Liver Cyst

The liver is commonly (60%) affected by hydatid disease. The disease is caused by *Echinococcus granulosus*, a tapeworm encountered in endemic countries such as the Mediterranean area (including North Africa, Spain, and Greece), the Middle East, Iran, the East of Europe, and in South American countries such as Argentina, Chile, and Uruguay. The disease has almost disappeared from other parts of the world such as Western Australia and New Zealand where sheep farming is common. The disease is seen all over the world because of increasing immigration and worldwide travel from high-risk regions. Humans are intermediate hosts after enteral ingestion of infective eggs from infested dogs. The parasite becomes encysted within the liver and develops a germinal membrane that is responsible for production of scolices, crystal clear hydatid fluid, and daughter cysts. With increasing-size, the host-compressed liver produces a reactive fibrous capsule encircling the hydatid liver cyst (HLC). The cyst is usually solitary and unilocular but may be multiple (25–30%) within the liver and the abdominal cavity or the lungs.

HLC is a slow-growing disease, remaining silent during a long clinical latency. Diagnosis is made on imaging and serologic studies, with a positive indirect hemagglutination test in more than 80% of the patients. A negative serological test does not rule out the diagnosis of echinococcosis, especially in patients with positive P1 or P2 erythrocytes serotypes. Eosinophilia is inconstant and liver tests are normal, except in cases of biliary complication. These lesions become symptomatic because of a space-occupying effect that produces abdominal pain or mass, allergic reactions, or more commonly, complications. HLC compresses progressively the surrounding intrahepatic parenchyma, blood vessels, and bile ducts. Biliary

complications are common (10–30%), and may be caused by rupture of the cyst content into the biliary tree which, in turn, is responsible for bile-staining intracystic fluid, abnormal liver tests, obstructive jaundice, or cholangitis. Other complications include cyst infection, compression of the portal system or the liver outflow (Budd-Chiari syndrome), rupture into the pleural, pericardial cavity or the bronchial tree, perforation into adjacent viscus (stomach, duodenum, small intestine), spontaneous, or posttraumatic rupture in the peritoneal cavity. This last complication is the least frequent but the most severe complication of hydatid disease, causing secondary peritoneal implantations that are difficult to eradicate.

Surgical treatment is usually recommended in all operable patients because of the often complicated clinical presentation of the disease, despite its benign nature. The purpose of surgical treatment is to eradicate completely the parasites, to obliterate the remaining cyst cavity, and to treat associated complications. The sonographic classification reported initially by Gharbi and colleagues and later modified by the World Health Organization aims to predict the functional state of hydatid disease and facilitate patient selection for treatment (Table 6.2).

Neoplastic Liver Cysts

Liver cystadenoma is a rare cystic tumor (representing <5% of hepatic cysts), with a strong tendency to recur after incomplete excision and undergo malignant transformation into cystadenocarcinoma. The disease occurs more often in middle-aged women. Macroscopically, the lesion is a single, usually large, multiloculated cyst, containing mucinous PAS-positive fluid. Irregularities or septations within the cyst wall are present. Microscopic examination reveals a single layer of mucin-secreting cuboidal epithelium with vacuolated cells and often polypoid or papillary projections are observed. Some mucinous liver cystadenomas harbor an ovarian-like mesenchymal stroma. Liver cystadenomas are premalignant lesions, with malignancy occurring almost exclusively in preexisting cystadenomas and potentially affecting the entire cyst epithelium

TABLE 6.2. Ultrasound (US) classification of hydatid liver cysts according to Gharbi et al. (1981) and WHO (2003).

Gharbi et al. (1981) classification	WHO (2003) classification	Ultrasound features	Parasitic activity status
—	CL	Pure fluid collection, unilocular, no cyst wall, signs not pathognomonic for hydatid cyst	Active
Type I	Type CE 1	Fluid collection with cyst wall, hydatid sand	Active
Type II	Type CE 2	Multivesicular fluid collection, cyst wall, "rosette-like"	Active
Type III	Type CE 3	Fluid collection with detached laminated membrane, "water-lily" sign, less round, decreased intracystic pressure	Transitional
Type IV	Type CE 4	Heterogeneous hypoechoic or hyperechoic cyst contents, high internal echoes, no daughter cysts	Inactive
Type V	Type CE 5	Thick calcified cyst wall, calcification partial to complete	Inactive

CL: cystic lesion; CE: *Echinococcus granulosus* cyst.

but more often involving only focal areas of malignant epithelial transformation. This feature explains why a needle biopsy can be falsely negative.

Liver cystadenoma is a slow-growing tumor. Symptoms are usually related to mass effects, including abdominal pain or discomfort. Extrahepatic or intrahepatic tumor compression may occur. Liver function tests are normal, but imaging studies and cyst fluid sampling are useful for diagnosis. Fine needle aspiration cytology (FNAC) examination and determination of CA-19-9 in the mucinous fluid can be suggestive of neoplastic liver cysts. Because of the malignant potential of liver cystadenoma, complete surgical excision is always indicated, even in asymptomatic patients. Indeed, partial excision exposes the patient to an almost constant risk of recurrence and further malignancy.

Other Uncommon Liver Cysts

Several liver diseases may appear cystic on imaging studies. Benign cystic conditions include posttraumatic liver hematoma or biloma, liver abscess, or cystic mesenchymal hamartoma. Previous history of right upper quadrant (RUQ) trauma directs the diagnosis to a traumatic origin. Additionally, the radiological aspect differs from that of true hepatic cysts, with the coexistence of nonliquefied liver hematoma forming a thick pseudocystic wall in cases of trauma. Liver abscess is suspected by the presence of high fever, chills, acute RUQ pain with elevated white cell count, and septicemia. Radiologically, liver abscesses have a thicker, more irregular wall than simple cysts and often contain debris which produces internal echoes. On computed tomography (CT) and magnetic resonance imaging (MRI), prominent perfusion abnormalities are often observed in the adjacent liver parenchyma. The history and clinical examination should help to differentiate abscesses and primary liver cysts. Mesenchymal hamartoma is characterized by a complex cystic-solid imaging appearance, thick wall, and some enhancing internal stromal components. Acquired malignant cystic diseases include complete or partial necrosis of large

primary tumors such as hepatocellular carcinoma or metastases from sarcoma, melanoma, lung, breast, and mucinous colorectal or neuroendocrine tumors. Central cystic degeneration or extensive tumor necrosis may result in a cyst-like appearance. However, with contrast-enhanced imaging, any central nonenhancing area is surrounded by peripheral nodular enhancement from viable tumor. Percutaneous biopsy of the thick cyst wall for histological examination will be helpful in obtaining a definitive diagnosis.

Characterization of Cystic Liver Lesions

An appropriate differential diagnosis among congenital, parasitic, and neoplastic cystic liver diseases is crucial, not only because of the differences in the natural disease history and malignant potential, but also for treatment planning. Characterization is based on patient's clinical history, blood samples, imaging studies, and often cyst-fluid analysis.

Clinical History

A history of travel from an endemic country favors a diagnosis of hydatid liver disease. A family history should be sought in patients suffering from PLD. A specific clinical background is encountered in case of traumatic liver pseudocyst and liver abscess. Otherwise, clinical history is of limited value in differentiating congenital from neoplastic liver cysts.

Blood Sampling

Serological tests, when positive, allow diagnosis of hydatid liver disease and an elevated serum Ca 19-9 is often encountered in overt or metastatic liver cystadenocarcinoma. Biological signs of infection and septicemia favor liver abscess. Elevated liver function tests are only predictive of biliary compression or intraductal migration of hydatid debris.

Imaging Studies

The typical radiological appearances are the cornerstone for characterizing cystic liver diseases. Percutaneous ultrasound (US) is the simplest and least expensive diagnostic imaging modality, but CT or MRI are increasingly used for differentiating hepatic cysts. Determining features for defining the cyst type include cyst number, density, septae and cyst wall thickness, and nodularity.

Congenital liver cysts appear as anechoic, hypodense avascular solitary lesions (Fig. 6.1), with an imperceptible or thin wall, without focal wall thickening or nodularity, without septation or intracystic formation and containing homogeneous fluid with strong posterior acoustic enhancement on US. Homogeneous cystic lesions with low signal intensity on T1-weighted images and high signal intensity on T2-weighted images are typical MRI features. It is usually considered that CLCs do not demonstrate septations except false septations due to contiguous CLCs. The intracystic fluid becomes heterogeneous in cases of hemorrhage or infection. It may

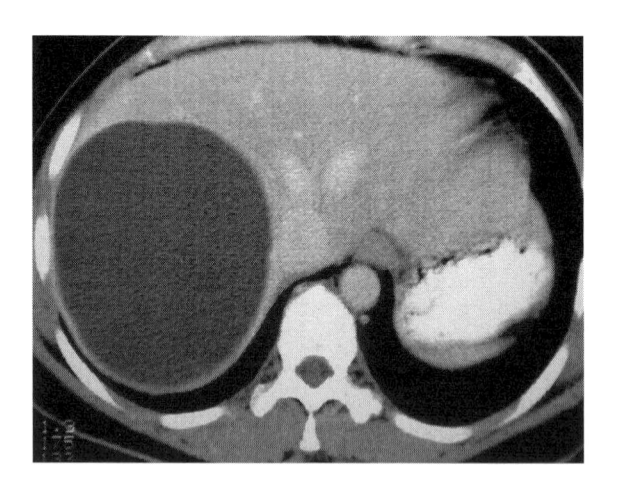

FIGURE 6.1. Uncomplicated congenital liver cyst: hypodense lesion, with a thin wall and a homogeneous cyst content.

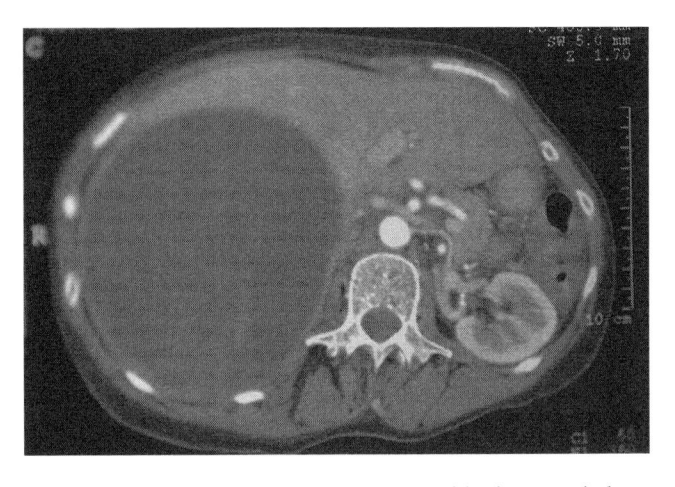

FIGURE 6.2. Congenital liver cyst complicated by intracystic hemorrhage: hyperdense cyst content due to blood clots.

contain echoes on US, demonstrate fluid layering or increased density on CT scan (Fig. 6.2) or appear hyperintense on T1-weighted images. The wall of a cyst complicated by hemorrhage or infection often becomes thick because of inflammation.

Hydatid liver cysts appear as a cystic lesion with a "double line" sign which reflects the pericyst and the laminate membrane of the cyst. Hydatid cysts contain homogeneous or heterogeneous fluid of variable density with internal daughter vesicles, "hydatid sand" and echogenic septa. Calcifications are observed in the hydatid cystic wall in 25% of the patients. CT and MRI demonstrate multiple septa and loculations, as well as daughter cysts (Fig. 6.3). The wall of the HLC is often thick and markedly hypointense on T2-weighted images because of their fibrous content. The radiological aspect of HLC is quite typical. However, some young, unilocular echinococcal liver cysts, with echo-free intracystic fluid (named type I in the ultrasound GHARBI classification) may simulate a simple CLC. Classical distinctive characteristics of simple and hydatid cysts of the liver are presented in Table 6.3. Additionally, hydatid disease may have been contracted in

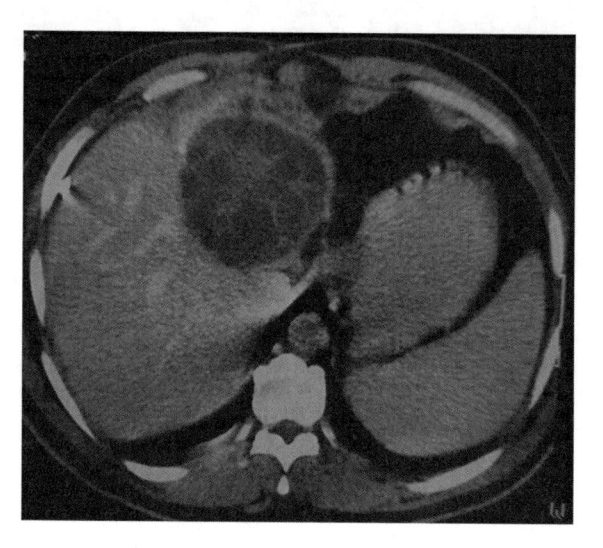

FIGURE 6.3. Hydatid liver cyst: heterogeneous cyst content with intracystic daughter cysts.

TABLE 6.3. Distinctive characteristics between congenital liver cysts and hydatid liver cysts.

	Congenital liver cyst	Hydatid liver cyst
History of stay in endemic countries	No	Yes
Blood samples		
Eosinophilia	Absent	Inconstant
Serological tests	Negative	Usually positive
Imaging features		
Septations	Absent	Common
Calcifications	Absent	Common
Split-wall	Absent	Common
Communication with biliary tree	Absent	Common

an area where this parasitic infection is not endemic and calcifications, septations, and split-wall may be absent.

Liver cystadenoma or cystadenocarcinoma appears as multiloculated lesions containing heterogeneous mucinous fluid and numerous intracystic internal septations due to intracystic papillary projections from a thick and irregular cystic wall. Internal septations, cystic wall, and mural nodules are enhanced after intravenous administration of contrast medium (Fig. 6.4). Sometimes, calcifications are seen in the septations and mural nodules. In cystadenocarcinoma, increased solid components within the cystic wall are observed. The distinctive characteristics of liver cystadenoma and CLC are listed in Table 6.4. In summary, any mural nodularity or irregular thickening, multiple septations, or a fluid level within a cystic mass are important criteria for an alternative diagnosis, such as hydatid or neoplastic cysts. However, despite the improvements in imaging techniques, the parasitic or neoplastic nature of an hepatic cyst still may be misdiagnosed, leading to inappropriate treatment exposing the patient to recurrence and reoperation.

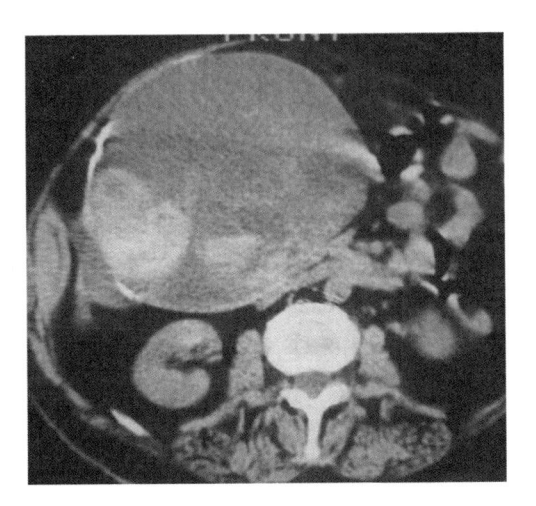

FIGURE 6.4. Liver cystadenocarcinoma: mural nodules within cyst wall with intracystic septations and heterogeneous cyst content.

TABLE 6.4. Distinctive characteristics between liver cystadenoma and congenital liver cysts (CLCs).

	Liver cystadenoma	Congenital liver cyst
Clinical history	Middle-aged women	All ages
Imaging studies		
Number of cysts	Unique	Unique or multiple
Presence of septations	Present	Absent
Presence of papillary projections	Common	Absent
Aspect of cystic fluid	Mucinous	Serous
Natural history		
Malignant transformation	Possible	Exceptional
Recurrence after partial excision	Common	Possible

Cyst-Fluid Evaluation

The features of cyst fluid are important in characterizing hepatic cysts: translucent fluid in congenital cysts, clear watery fluid in echinococcal cysts, and blood or mucoid contents in neoplastic cysts. However, in CLC complicated by bleeding or infection, the aspect of cyst fluid is brownish or bloody and may be confused with the one of neoplastic cysts. Percutaneous cystic aspiration with cytology and assays for carcinoembryogenic antigen (CEA) and CA-19-9 of the cystic fluid are useful in differentiating cystic hepatic neoplasms. However, when a resectable liver cystadenocarcinoma is suspected on imaging, fine needle aspiration biopsy should be avoided to prevent tumor seeding. Additionally, reactional changes to the cyst wall from bleeding or infection may also be confusing. Thus, great attention should still be paid to any

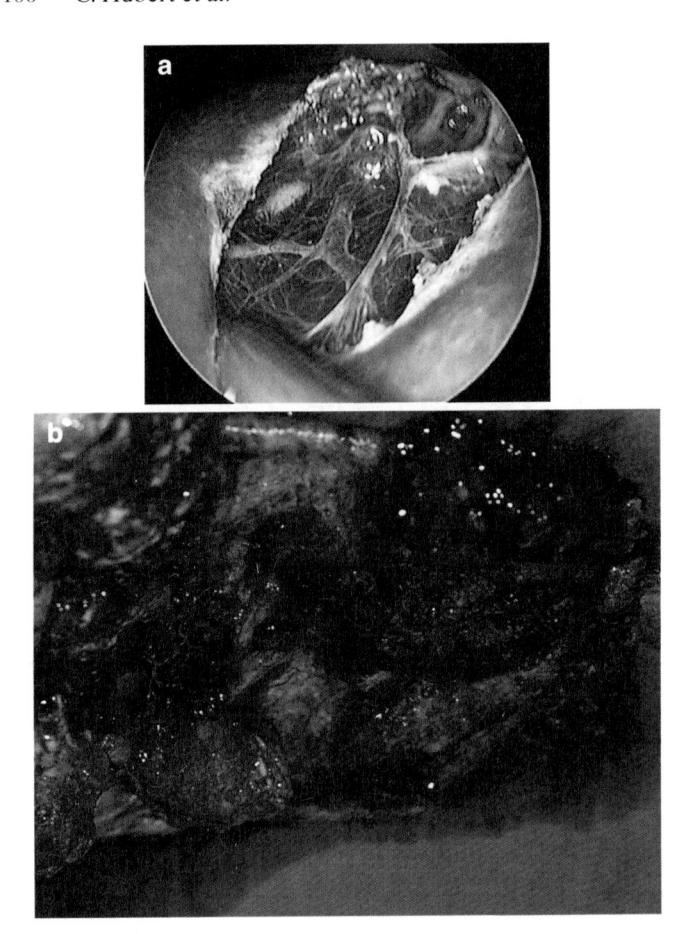

FIGURE 6.5. Macroscopic appearance of inner cyst wall at surgical exploration. (a) Typical appearance of a congenital liver cyst: thin transparent cyst wall allowing visualization of liver parenchyma and vessels. (b) Typical features of liver cystadenocarcinoma: thick cyst wall with papillary polypoid projections, vegetations and mucoid fluid within the cyst.

unusual cystic fluid appearances and to careful inspection of the inner aspect of the cyst wall to exclude irregular and nodular areas (Fig. 6.5). Such abnormalities should prompt the undertaking of multiple biopsies and frozen section

examination to rule out a neoplastic liver cyst. Specimens should be of adequate size and several biopsies, particularly from areas of thickening or irregularity in the cyst wall, may be necessary. The importance of these issues is well illustrated by the series of Wellwood et al. in which the nature of two malignant cysts was not recognized during operation.

Treatment

Treatment options should be tailored to the type of liver cyst, and thus preoperative differentiation and correct preoperative diagnosis is crucial. The management of cystic liver diseases has recently benefited from progress in interventional radiology and laparoscopic surgery.

Congenital Liver Cysts

When indicated, treatment options for CLC include surgery or percutaneous ablative techniques. At present, no comparative study evaluating these approaches has been reported. A treatment algorithm for CLC is detailed in Fig. 6.6. The choice of treatment should be guided by cyst number and intrahepatic location, coexistent cyst complications, and patient risk factors. Surgical treatment includes fenestration techniques, which are usually performed through a laparoscopic approach that has become the gold standard minimally invasive surgical option. Large, superficial, accessible cysts on the liver surface (the cyst appearance should be carefully inspected on preoperative CT) and located in the anterior liver segments 2–6 are ideal indications for a laparoscopic approach. On the contrary, posterior or deep-sited cysts are difficult to approach laparoscopically. These last patients may be good candidates for percutaneous alcohol sclerotherapy or for an open surgical approach. Finally, CLC located in segment VIII are more prone to early cyst recurrence after a deroofing technique because the residual cyst cavity is immediately covered by the diaphragm unless an in situ omentoplasty is employed

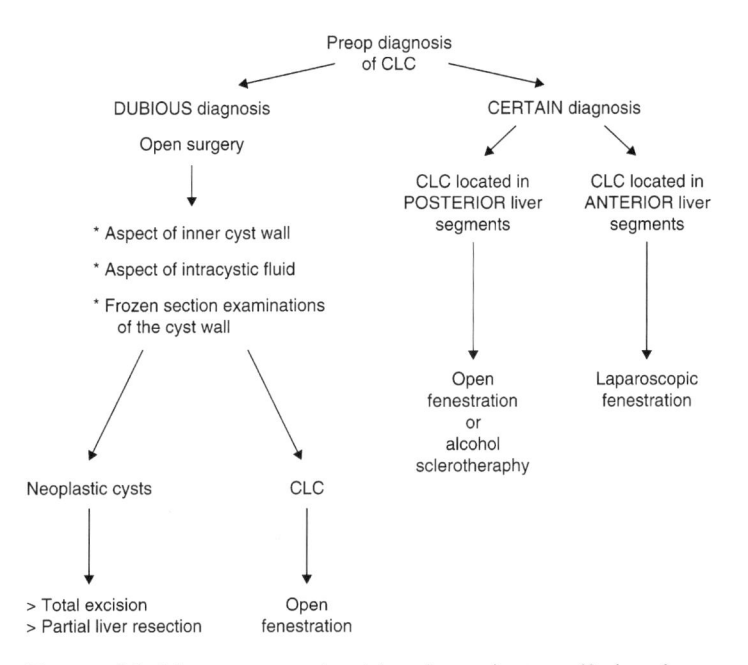

FIGURE 6.6. Management algorithm in patients suffering from congenital liver cysts (CLCs).

to obliterate the cystic cavity. Appropriate and meticulous surgical techniques should be used to achieve good results. These include a wide deroofing technique using harmonic shears, careful preservation of surrounding liver parenchyma to avoid bleeding, careful inspection of the fenestrated cyst wall for possible bile leakage during the procedure, and ablation of the cyst lining epithelium of the residual cystic cavity by the use of Argon Beam Coagulator. When using strict selection of patients and appropriate surgical techniques, definite success rate exceeding 90% can be obtained with no reported mortality and a complication rate <10–15%. An open procedure or conversion during laparoscopic approaches should be reserved to atypical CLC with a dubious preoperative diagnosis or when a neoplastic cyst cannot be ruled out during surgical exploration. Percutaneous cyst sclerotherapy with alcohol under US or CT guidance has been reported as

another minimally invasive approach for treating CLC. While simple cyst aspiration is always associated with cyst recurrence, alcohol sclerotherapy is a very efficient technique. Repeat sessions of interventional procedures are usually needed with large cysts. However, a cystogram should be performed before alcohol sclerotherapy to exclude biliary communication, which is a contraindication for the technique. Successful results are achieved in 70–90% of patients, with no mortality and very low morbidity (<10%). Late cyst recurrence occurs in 0–15%.

Polycystic Liver Disease

The purpose of any treatment option is to reduce significantly (or to replace) the mass effect of the huge polycystic liver with minimal morbidity in order to achieve long-term relief of symptoms and to improve the patient's quality of life. Currently, the most appropriate therapeutic approach for PLD remains controversial and rests between laparoscopic or open fenestration approaches (2), open partial liver resection (8), and liver transplantation. A treatment algorithm for PLD patients is detailed in Fig. 6.7. Type I PLD should be considered for a laparoscopic approach, if dominant liver cysts are superficial and accessible. The fenestration technique is the same as that used for treating CLC. Percutaneous alcohol sclerotherapy should be reserved for high-risk patients, to contraindications of a laparoscopic approach of CLC, or for selective ablation of a deep-sited compressive dominant hepatic cyst.

The surgical management of type II PLD is more controversial, including open fenestration techniques with or without partial liver resection. Very few patients can be approached laparoscopically and only if dominant hepatic cysts are located in the anterior liver segments. The concept of fenestration is to unroof as many cysts as possible, starting from the superficial and then, stepwise, opening the deep-sited cysts, taking great care to avoid vascular and biliary tract injuries within the cystic septa. If two or more adjacent liver

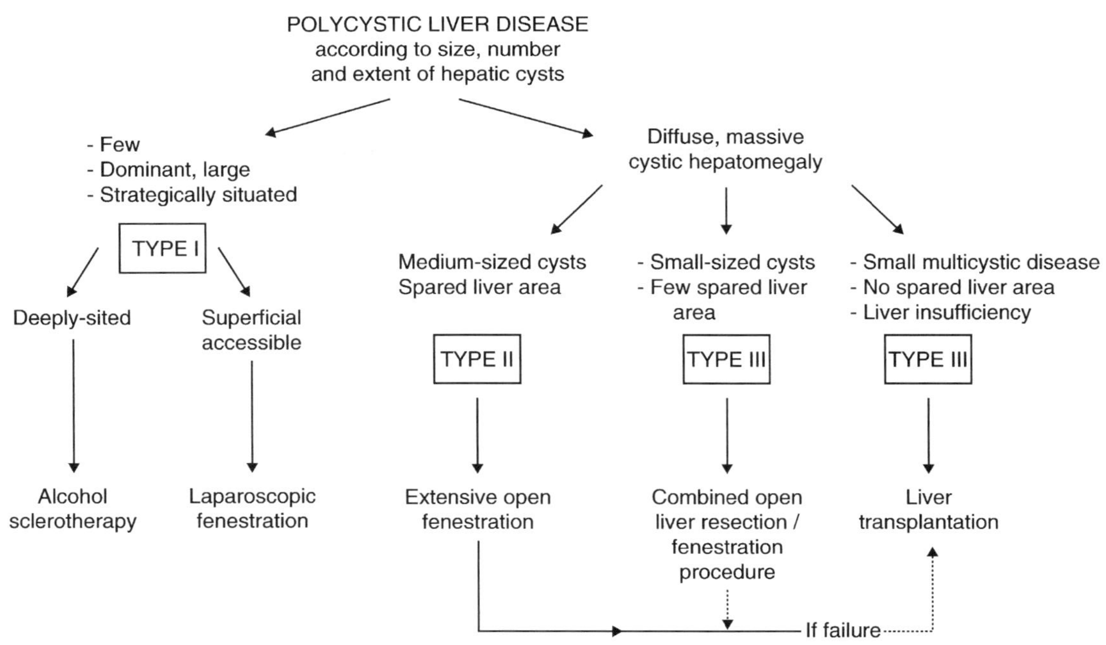

FIGURE 6.7. Strategy for treatment of highly symptomatic patients with polycystic liver disease.

segments are spared by the disease, combined liver resection/ fenestration can be chosen. In the limited reported clinical experience with open fenestration techniques in patients with PLD, the mortality was low (1–5%), but the complication rate was significant (40–50%), including ascites (50–70%) and biliary leaks. The purpose of liver resection is to achieve long-term relief from symptoms by inducing a significant reduction in the volume of massive cystic hepatomegaly. In the limited reported clinical experience, the mortality was 5–10% and the complication rate was not insignificant (50–60%).

Liver transplantation should be considered for diffuse forms of type III PLD without any segmental sparing as well as for patients with liver insufficiency, after recurrence following initial liver resection or in cases of end-stage PKD, combining in such cases, liver and kidney transplantation. Due to the complicated presentation of this benign disease and the significant complication rates of all types of surgical treatments of these difficult patients, each case must be discussed with a multidisciplinary team approach, including hepatologists, nephrologists, and liver and transplant surgeons.

Hydatid Liver Cysts

Until recently, only surgical treatment was effective for HLC. With the advent of percutaneous injection of scolicidal agents and laparoscopic surgery, the treatment strategy for echinococcal liver cysts has been challenged. The treatment algorithm for HDL is given in Fig. 6.8, according to the WHO disease classification which is a useful guide to the treatment decision-making process. Indications for surgery include large cysts with multiple daughter cysts, superficial liver cysts prone to rupture, infected cysts, cysts communicating with the biliary tree, cysts compressing adjacent organs, and extrahepatic cysts. Contraindications for surgery include elderly and high-risk patients, pregnancy, multiple deep-sited intraparenchymal cysts which are difficult to access, dead cysts, totally calcified cysts, and very small cysts.

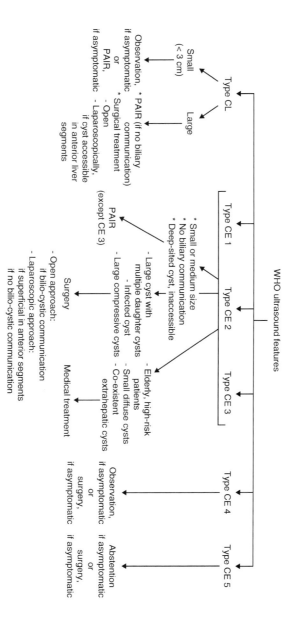

FIGURE 6.8. Strategy for treatment of hydatid liver cysts.

The objectives of *operative management of HDL* include adequate exposure of the cyst, safe cyst decompression with prevention of intraperitoneal spillage, sterilization, and complete removal of parasitic cystic content, management of cysto-biliary communications, management of the residual cavity, and finally the detection and treatment of other abdominal lesions. Meticulous protection of the peritoneal cavity from spillage is crucial. When approached through a laparotomy, the operation begins by placing packs with hypertonic solution around the liver to absorb any inadvertent spillage of cyst content during the procedure. The cyst is decompressed partially with a Trocar and the cyst content is aspirated as much as possible. Then the scolicidal agent is instilled within the cyst to sterilize the parasite. Formalin is no longer used for sterilization of HDL content, due to the risk of biliary damage when a cyst-biliary communication exists. The most commonly used scolicidal agent is 20% hypertonic saline solution. Once the cyst is opened and deroofed, the germinal membrane and residual daughter cysts are removed and the inner host capsule is carefully inspected to exclude any biliary fistula. A methylene blue test is employed by cystic duct injection to detect occult fistula. Preoperative detection and treatment of cysto-biliary communications is essential to avoid occasional severe postoperative complications. If the bile duct is obstructed by hydatid material, surgical or endoscopic common bile duct clearance is performed with external or internal biliary drainage, associated with direct suture of the cysto-biliary fistula within the cystic cavity. In the few instances where the HDL communicates with a major hilar bile duct, a Roux-en-Y cysto-jejunostomy or an intracystic hepatico-jejunostomy may be necessary. Finally, the residual cystic cavity is obliterated by omentoplasty. Peritoneal drainage of the cystic cavity is always indicated.

More radical procedures can be used to manage the residual cyst cavity such as cysto-pericystectomy, by removing partially or completely the host-derived fibrous pericyst. This procedure is technically more demanding, but has the main advantage of avoiding entirely a residual cystic cavity and

preventing disease recurrence. However, when HDL is closely adjacent or adherent to major intrahepatic vessels or biliary radicles, partial pericystectomy should be performed. If small parts of the pericyst are left in place, there is a risk of bile leak and sepsis. Formal liver resection is rarely indicated except in cases of severe parenchymal destruction. Surgical treatment of the echinococcal cyst carries a mortality rate of 1–4% and a complication rate of 20–30%. The most frequent postoperative complications are overlooked cysto-biliary communications or hydatid debris in the common bile duct, cyst cavity infection, pleuro-pulmonary complications and wound infection. Postoperative bile collection or chronic biliary fistula should be managed by endoscopic sphincterotomy and stenting. The long-term recurrence rate is approximately 5–10%. Cyst growth appears to be the best imaging marker for diagnosing locally recurrent disease during follow-up.

Laparoscopic management of HDL has been recently advocated as being able to fill all the objectives of surgical disease treatment. However, the limited area for surgical manipulation and the difficulty in controlling spillage during puncture and decompression are disadvantages of this approach. Treatment of biliary communication is also difficult by laparoscopic means and may lead to conversion to an open approach. Indications of laparoscopic surgery include type CE 1–3 HDL in an accessible location. Exclusion criteria for laparoscopic management include preoperatively anticipated biliary communication, deep intra-parenchymal cysts, a posterior inaccessible cyst, multiple (> 3) cysts, and cysts with thick and calcified walls. Conversion to open laparotomy is indicated in cases of unsafe exposure, unsatisfactory access, intraoperative bleeding, and spillage in the peritoneal cavity or intrabiliary cyst rupture. Postoperative morbidity in laparoscopic series is reported to be 8–25% (open series: 12–63%) with treatment-related mortality in almost 0%. The rate of short-term recurrence following laparoscopic treatment of HDL is reported to be 0–9%.

Percutaneous aspiration injection reaspiration (PAIR) technique, under US or CT guidance, is gaining acceptance as a minimally invasive treatment of this benign disease, because

of its low morbidity and easy applicability, but selection of patients is of paramount importance. Percutaneous treatment is indicated for CE type 1 and 2 HDL, some groups of CE type 3 that do not contain solid material, suspect fluid collections (CL), and in patients with univesicular recurrent cysts and infected hydatid cysts. Contraindications include subgroups of CE types 3 and 4 and cysts that have ruptured into the biliary tree or the peritoneal cavity. There is a theoretical risk of dissemination, peritoneal spillage, and anaphylactic shock (0.1–0.2%). However, the mortality rate (0.9–2.5%) and the complication rate (15–40%) are low.

Medical treatment with Mebendazole or Albendazole is currently indicated for inoperable patients, multiple intra-abdominal, or combined intra-and extra-abdominal disease, multiple small liver cysts, and small central hydatid cysts requiring major hepatectomy as an alternative treatment procedure. Its use can be considered in the prevention and management of secondary hydatidosis, management of recurrent disease, in combination with surgery and interventional radiology, for pulmonary hydatid disease and for hydatid diseases in bones. A prospective controlled trial has demonstrated the efficacy of preoperative administration of Albendazole in preparation to surgery and may obviate the need for scolicidal agents with their inherent risks. Side effects of Mebendazole include nausea, abdominal discomfort, and occasional vomiting but are rarely serious. Hepatotoxicity, alopecia, and leucopenia have also been reported. Chemotherapy is contraindicated in large liver cysts, cysts with multiple septa-division, honeycomb-like cysts, superficial cysts prone to rupture, infected cysts, inactive cysts, calcified cysts, coexistent severe chronic liver diseases, bone marrow depression, and pregnancy.

Neoplastic Cysts

Complete excision of neoplastic liver cysts is required. Due to the potential for malignancy, partial excision exposes the patient to the risk of recurrence and further malignancy. Benign

liver cystadenoma may be enucleated but the diagnosis of malignant transformation can only be made on final pathological examination. Radical liver resection should thus be preferred with adequate tumor-free margins. Long-term survival has only been reported after complete resection of neoplastic liver cysts.

Selected Readings

Devernis Ch, Delis S, Avgerinos C, et al. (2005) Changing concepts in the management of liver hydatic disease. J Gastrointest Surg 9:869–877

Gharbi H, Hassine W, Brauner MW, et al. (1981) Ultrasound examination of the hydatid liver. Radiology 139:459–463

Gigot JF, Jadoul P, Que F, et al. (1997) Adult polycystic liver disease: is fenestration the most adequate operation for long-term management? Ann Surg 225:286–294

Gigot JF, Métairie S, Etienne J, et al. (2001) The surgical management of congenital liver cysts: the need for a tailored approach with appropriate patient selection and proper surgical technique. Surg Endosc 15:357–363

Gil-Grande LA, Rodriguez-Caabeiro F, Prieto JG, et al. (1993) Randomized controlled trial of efficacy of albendazole in intraabdominal hydatid disease. Lancet 342:1269–1272

Horsmans Y, Laka A, Gigot JF, et al. (1996) Serum and cyst fluid CA 19.9 determinations as a diagnostic help in liver cysts of uncertain nature. Liver 16:255–257

Ishak KG, Willis GW, Cummins SD, et al. (1977) Biliary cystadenoma and cystadenocarcinoma. Report of 14 cases and review of the literature. Cancer 38:322–338

Que F, Nagorney DM, Gross JB, et al. (1995) Liver resection and cyst fenestration in the treatment of severe polycystic liver disease. Gastroenterology 108:487–494

Wellwood JM, Madara JL, Cady B, et al. (1978) Large intrahepatic cysts and pseudocysts: pitfalls in diagnosis and treatment. Am J Surg 135:57–64

WHO Informal Working Group on Echinococcosis (2003) International classification of ultrasound images in cystic echonococcosis for application in clinical and field epidemiological settings. Acta Trop 85:253–261

7
Liver Transplantation for Budd-Chiari Syndrome

François Durand and Jacques Belghiti

Pearls and Pitfalls

- Budd-Chiari syndrome is almost always associated with underlying prothrombotic conditions such as myeloproliferative disorders.
- In cases where Budd-Chiari syndrome first presents with acute liver failure (rare presentation), emergency transplantation is the safest approach unless TIPS (trans-jugular insertion of a portosystemic shunt) can be undertaken in specialist centers.
- In patients with a chronic presentation, of refractory ascites, that cannot be improved by medical management or TIPS, represents the main indication for transplantation. Chronic encephalopathy following TIPS or surgical portosystemic shunt may also be an indication for transplantation.
- Early mortality following surgical portosystemic shunt is not significantly lower than that of transplantation; however, transplantation offers better long term survival.
- Patients with an underlying prothrombotic state, which is not reversed by transplantation should receive long-term anticoagulation. Vitamin K antagonists are standard therapy.

K.I. Bland et al. (eds.), *Liver and Biliary Surgery*,
DOI 10.1007/978-1-84996-429-6_7,
© Springer-Verlag London Limited 2011

- TIPS misplacement can produce major technical difficulties during transplantation. When there is a potential indication for transplantation, it is strongly recommended that extension of the shunt over the ostium of the hepatic veins or within the main portal vein is avoided.
- Concomitant portal and mesenteric vein thrombosis is usually considered a contraindication for transplantation.
- Mortality following transplantation for Budd-Chiari syndrome mainly occurs during the first 3 months after the procedure.

Introduction

Budd-Chiari syndrome is a rare condition defined as hepatic outflow obstruction at any level from the small hepatic veins to the junction of the inferior vena cava and the right atrium, regardless of the cause of obstruction. In most cases, outflow obstruction results from obliterative thrombosis involving main (right, median and left) through to small hepatic vein branches. In rare instances, hepatic outflow obstruction may result from a membranous web of the inferior vena cava, extrinsic compression or even from intraluminal invasion by a tumor.

Although in some patients, the first manifestation can be acute with rapidly progressive liver failure, Budd-Chiari syndrome is a chronic liver disease. Thrombosis does not abruptly involve all hepatic vein branches but rather progresses over time, involving an increasing number of vessels. Chronic hepatic outflow obstruction results in sinusoidal dilatation, congestion and hepatocyte necrosis and predominates in the central areas of the hepatic lobules. Centrilobular fibrosis progresses over time and nodular regenerative changes result. A frequent finding is superimposed thrombosis of intrahepatic small to middle size portal veins.

More than 70% of patients with hepatic vein thrombosis are found to have an underlying prothrombotic state consisting of a myeloproliferative disorder and/or coagulation disorder. The list of the underlying prothrombotic states in patients with Budd-Chiari syndrome are shown in Table 7.1.

TABLE 7.1. Prothrombotic states in patients with Budd-Chiari syndrome and reversibility with transplantation.

Predisposing factor	Reversibility with transplantation
Myeloproliferative disorders	
• Polycythemia vera	No
• Essential thrombocythemia	No
• Others rare disorders	No
Coagulation disorders	
• Factor V Leiden mutation	Yes
• Protein C deficiency	Yes
• Protein S deficiency	Yes
• Antithrombin deficiency	Yes
• Plasminogen deficiency	Yes
• Factor II mutation	Yes
• Antiphospholipid syndrome	No
Paroxysmal nocturnal hemoglobinuria	No
Behçet's disease	No
Pregnancy	–

Natural History and Prognosis of Budd-Chiari Syndrome

The natural history of Budd-Chiari syndrome varies from patient to patient. Most patients, experience complications related to portal hypertension such as ascites or variceal bleeding before 40 years of age. In some patients, the disease first manifests as massive liver cell necrosis and liver failure, probably as a consequence of an abrupt extension of thrombosis to previously preserved hepatic vein branches or collaterals. In this latter group, the prognosis is considered to be especially poor and when encephalopathy is present.

After a first episode of decompensation, the progression of the disease is variable. It is generally easy to prevent

recurrence of variceal bleeding with beta-blockers or endoscopic elastic band ligation. In some patients, ascites is controlled with standard therapy, however, others develop refractory ascites with subsequent malnutrition and muscular atrophy. Other complications such as liver insufficiency, jaundice and encephalopathy may occur in parallel with ascites.

Determining the prognosis for Budd-Chiari syndrome is difficult. Besides the variability in the natural history, the outcome is influenced markedly by the various therapeutic interventions and the experience and skilled use of these by the treating center. It has been shown that the prognosis is influenced significantly by the independent variables of encephalopathy, ascites, INR and serum bilirubin. A prognostic score has been derived to allow identification of three groups of increasing severity risk (Table 7.2). The presence of portal vein thrombosis is associated significantly with a poor outcome. Eventually, some patients may develop hepatocellular carcinoma (HCC) although its incidence is much lower than in patients with cirrhosis of other origin.

Overall, not all patients, even those with an "acute-like" presentation, have a poor prognosis in the short and medium term. Reliable prognostic indexes, which take into account the most recent therapeutic options (TIPS in particular) and the causative disease are lacking.

TABLE 7.2. Prognosis of Budd-Chiari syndrome according to risk score: (1.27 encephalopathy + 1.04 ascites + 0.72 INR + 0.004 bilirubin [μmol/l])[a] (Murad et al., 2004).

Group	Risk score	5-year survival	95% confidence interval
1	0 to 1.1	89%	79%–99%
2	1.1 to 1.5	74%	65%–83%
3	Over 1.5	42%	28%–56%

[a]Encephalopathy and ascites are scored 0 if absent and 1 if present; INR is scored 0 if lower than 2.3 and 1 if greater than 2.3.

Treatments other than Transplantation

The treatment of patients with symptomatic Budd-Chiari syndrome has two objectives; namely, to prevent further thrombosis and to achieve liver decompression.

Lifelong anticoagulation is the key in preventing further extension of thrombosis, either to patent accessory hepatic veins (or collaterals) or to the portal vein where blood flow may be slowed or even reversed. Vitamin K-antagonists (warfarin and derivates) represent the gold standard for long-term anticoagulation. In the long term, patients with polycythemia vera or essential thrombophilia may benefit from hydroxyurea to reduce hematocrit or platelet count. It has yet to be determined whether antiplatelet treatment is as effective or even superior to vitamin K antagonists in those patients with essential thrombophilia.

For years, surgical portosystemic shunting has been the reference procedure for achieving liver decompression in patients who remain symptomatic despite medical management. It has been shown that surgical shunting improves survival for patients with Budd-Chiari syndrome of intermediate severity (class 2, Table 7.2). In contrast, there is no clear benefit for patients with mild (class 1) or high severity (class 3) compared to medical management alone. Surgery is limited by in-hospital mortality, which is as high as 20% and a 30% rate of shunt dysfunction, due to thrombosis or stenosis in particular. This morbidity and mortality has been an incentive for developing percutaneous techniques (stenting and TIPS) as an alternative to surgery. Even in cases of complete obstruction of the hepatic veins, it is generally possible to insert a TIPS by trans-hepatic puncture through a hepatic vein stump, towards the right branch of the portal vein. Recent studies suggest that the morbidity is lower than that of surgical shunt and that sustained improvement can be achieved. However, long term results have not been well assessed.

Indications and Timing for Liver Transplantation

Liver transplantation, being a demanding procedure, is only justified in patients with severe complications, which are refractory or not amenable to other therapeutic options except by a surgical shunt. Surgical shunt carries early mortality and morbidity risks equal to or even greater than transplantation but with poorer long term results. Therefore, transplantation should be considered as a first line option in patients who otherwise could be potential candidates for surgical shunt.

Indications differ according to which patients have an acute or chronic presentation. In patients with an acute presentation, emergency transplantation may be justified by the occurrence of acute liver failure. Indeed, patients with high serum transaminases (over 10 times the upper limit of normal), an associated severe decrease in coagulation factors and who eventually develop encephalopathy have an especially poor prognosis with conventional therapy. "Rescue" TIPS possibly represents an alternative to transplantation in patients with acute liver failure and successful cases with longstanding improvement have been reported. However, TIPS placement is much more demanding in Budd-Chiari syndrome than in patients with cirrhosis. Only in a few centers are there sufficient technical skill in TIPS to allow the use of this technique in an emergency setting. Nonetheless, if TIPS placement is impossible due to technical reasons or if the patient continues to deteriorate despite a patent TIPS, emergency transplantation should be performed. In our experience, patients with an acute-like presentation and a failure in TIPS placement rapidly develop severe acidosis and multiorgan failure. Therefore, whatever the initial option that might be considered, acute liver failure in the context of Budd-Chiari syndrome should be managed preferably in a center where there is access to emergency transplantation.

In patients with a chronic presentation, refractory ascites and poor nutritional status resistant to nonsurgical therapeutic options including TIPS, represent the main indications for

transplantation. Similarly, patients with repeated episodes of hepatic encephalopathy or chronic encephalopathy following a surgical shunt or TIPS should be listed for transplantation. Patients with chronic encephalopathy should be transplanted within 3 to 6 months since neurological changes secondary to longstanding encephalopathy may not be fully reversible after transplantation. HCC is an extremely uncommon complication of Budd-Chiari syndrome but, on theoretical grounds, guidelines for transplantation should be identical to those patients with cirrhosis and HCC; a single nodule less than 5 cm or 2 or 3 nodules each less than 3 cm. However, many patients with chronic Budd-Chiari syndrome have large, hypervascular, regenerative nodules, with features indistinguishable from those of HCC. Therefore, the identification of one or several malignant nodules among a number of regenerative nodules may be impossible. Patients with large tumors at the time of diagnosis are unlikely to benefit from transplantation due to the high risk of tumor recurrence. Till date, it has been impossible to propose practical guidelines to screen for HCC and make a decision for transplantation in the setting of Budd-Chiari syndrome.

Irrespective of whether the initial presentation is acute or chronic, a stepwise therapeutic approach seems appropriate, beginning with less invasive options with progression to a more aggressive approach when there is insufficient response or lack of success. Liver transplantation represents the most aggressive therapeutic option, but it has demonstrated good long term results with an excellent quality of life in most cases.

Contraindications for Transplantation

Relative and absolute contraindications for transplantation may be related to the underlying causative disease of the Budd-Chiari syndrome or most frequently due to technical limitations.

Some patients with paroxysmal nocturnal hemoglobinuria may not be candidates for transplantation due to the poor prognosis of their underlying disease. Conversely, obvious

or latent myeloproliferative disorders do not represent contraindications for transplantation since prognosis is good and does not preclude long term survival after surgery. Most inherited coagulation disorders result from the reduced synthesis of normal coagulation factors or from deficient coagulation factors by the native liver. These disorders are corrected by liver transplantation and do not represent a contraindication (Table 7.1). Acquired disorders such as the antiphospholipid syndrome, in contrast, are not reversed by transplantation. However, long term anticoagulation following surgery is likely to prevent recurrence of thrombosis. Budd-Chiari syndrome due to underlying malignancy has to be recognized because it represents a definitive contraindication.

Portal vein thrombosis is observed in up to 20% of patients with Budd-Chiari syndrome. Transplantation can be considered in such cases since restoration of portal blood flow may be successful after thrombectomy. Conversely, an organized thrombus extending to splenic and mesenteric veins represents a contraindication since portal perfusion of the graft cannot be achieved. In such patients, caval transposition has been proposed as an alternative technique since the donor's portal vein can be perfused via a porto-caval anastomosis. Unfortunately, the results of this technique have been dismal due to the high operative risk and the persistence of portal hypertension.

Technical Aspects

The widely adopted "piggy back technique" (preservation of the native inferior vena cava with by end-to-side caval anastomosis) may be difficult to perform in patients with Budd-Chiari syndrome. Firstly, the caudate lobe is markedly enlarged and dense adhesions are frequent adjacent to the suprahepatic vena cava. Secondly, thrombotic changes commonly involve the inferior vena cava, precluding end-toside anastomosis. Furthermore, most patients with Budd-Chiari have prominent collateral vessels due to marked portal hypertension, which is a significant source of blood loss. As a

consequence of the compression of the enlarged caudate lobe, the pressure is usually higher in the inferior than in superior vena cava. The pressure gradient between the portal vein and the inferior vena cava is reduced, precluding the hemodynamic effect of a porto-caval shunt. In such cases, early institution of venovenous bypass is recommended with the return canula sited in the territory of the superior vena cava since this is likely to be functionally superior to temporary porto-caval anastomosis. After total clamping, the native liver and retrohepatic vena cava can be removed *en bloc*, followed by the implantation of the graft using an end-to-end caval anastomosis. This "standard" technique is also applicable in patients with organized thrombus of the retrohepatic vena cava that is not amenable thrombectomy.

Previous end-to-side porta-caval or meso-caval shunts should be dissected carefully. Previous meso-atrial shunts are more difficult to deal with and should obviously be ligated before graft reperfusion to ensure adequate portal perfusion. As indicated previously, an increasing number of patients have had TIPS placement before transplantation. If there is proximal extension of the shunt over the junction between the ostium of the hepatic veins, it can be impossible to free the TIPS or stent from the wall of inferior vena cava and to perform partial clamping of the ostium. With distal extension to the confluence of the mesenteric and splenic vein, it may be similarly difficult to free the TIPS from the main portal vein. Either proximal or distal extension precludes the use of split or living donor grafts. Occasionally, some patients have undergone retrohepatic inferior vena cava stenting prior to transplantation. Stent extension within the right atrium can make it impossible to free or clamp the suprahepatic inferior vena cava.

Post Transplantation Management

Massive post operative ascites seems to be more frequent in patients with Budd-Chiari syndrome than in those with cirrhosis secondary to parenchymal diseases. The presence of

refractory ascites before transplantation predicts persistent ascites after the procedure. However, there is no evidence that Budd-Chiari syndrome has a specific impact but careful management of fluid losses is often needed within the first weeks.

Immunosuppression regimens do not differ from those of other transplanted patients but it is generally recommended that patients with myeloproliferative disorders receive anti-coagulation indefinitely, as the risk of hepatic artery thrombosis is higher than that of venous thrombosis. Anticoagulation is based on heparin or low molecular weight-heparin within the first few weeks followed by vitamin K antagonists with a target INR (International Normalized Ratio) of 1.5:3. Bleeding complications after transplantation seem relatively uncommon and are reported as less than 10%. As shown in Table 7.1, most inherited coagulation disorders are reversed by liver transplantation. However, there is lack of clear evidence that patients with Budd-Chiari syndrome due to coagulation disorders are no longer at increased risk of thrombosis after transplantation. Since Budd-Chiari syndrome is more likely to be due to the combination of several prothrombotic states, longstanding anticoagulation is recommended generally in this population.

In patients with underlying myeloproliferative disorders, a combination consisting of hydroxyurea and anti-platelet agents has been proposed as an alternative to long term anti-vitamin K therapy but their precise role is not yet determined.

Results of Liver Transplantation

Since Budd-Chiari syndrome is a rare condition, most publications on liver transplantation include a limited number of patients (Table 7.3). The largest series at the present time, comes from a multicenter European study of 248 patients. This series shows that 5-year probability of survival approaches 70%. Early mortality (within the first 3 months) accounted for more than 70% of the post transplantation deaths, similar

TABLE 7.3. Survival after transplantation for Budd-Chiari syndrome.

Author/reference	Year	Patients	Survival		
			1-year	3-year	5-year
Halff et al. 1990	1990	23	69%	45%	45%
Jamieson et al. 1991	1991	26	69%	69%	50%
Shaked et al. 1992	1992	14	86%	76%	–
Srinivasan et al. 2002	2002	19	95%	95%	95%
Ulrich et al. 2002	2002	27	–	–	87%
Mentha et al. 2006	2006	248	76%	–	71%

to that observed in patients transplanted for end-stage cirrhosis and poor nutritional status. Impaired renal function prior to transplantation and a past history of shunt have been found to be predictive of post transplantation mortality. One year survival may be as low as 60% in patients with a serum creatinine greater than 160 µmol/L before transplantation; suggesting that transplantation might be better performed before the occurrence of renal failure. The main causes of early mortality include sepsis, multiple organ failure and graft loss from hepatic artery thrombosis.

Recurrence of Budd-Chiari occurs in less than 2% of cases. Portal vein thrombosis is also uncommon although the reported incidence of 7% appears higher than in patients transplanted for other chronic liver diseases. However, patients with persistent prothrombotic disorders are more likely to develop complex vascular diseases of liver graft in the long term (for e.g. nodular regenerative hyperplasia-like syndrome) and need to be investigated.

The prognosis of most myeloproliferative disorders associated with Budd-Chiari syndrome is good in the long term. The progression of these disorders does not seem to affect the results of transplantation, at least within the first 5–10 years. However, it can be suspected that the proper course of myeloproliferative disorders could have a deleterious impact in the very long term.

Organ Allocation and Prioritization

Previously asymptomatic patients presenting with acute liver failure secondary to Budd-Chiari syndrome have an especially poor prognosis, the course of the disease being comparable to that of acute liver failure due to other causes. It is accepted generally that if these patients meet the criteria for transplantation, they should be placed on an emergency list (UNOS status 1A).

In patients with a chronic presentation, an unresolved issue is whether MELD (Model End-Stage Liver Disease) score is appropriate for organ allocation. MELD which relies on serum bilirubin, INR and creatinine, is a robust marker of mortality within 3 months in cirrhotic patients. However, there are several limitations regarding the use of this score in Budd-Chiari syndrome. Firstly, the MELD score variables are different from the independent prognostic markers, encephalopathy, ascites, INR and bilirubin (Table 7.2) identified in Budd-Chiari patients. Secondly, refractory ascites is a leading indication for transplantation in a Budd-Chiari syndrome. As shown previously, MELD underscores the disease severity in a number of patients with refractory ascites and a low serum sodium seems to be an important prognostic marker in this particular population. Thirdly, most patients with Budd-Chiari syndrome are placed on vitamin K antagonists thereby rendering the use of INR redundant. On the other hand, there is no clear evidence that for a given MELD score (and taking into account increased INR on vitamin K antagonists), patients with Budd-Chiari syndrome have an increased mortality risk when listed for transplantation. Therefore, up until the present, no specific score and no "extra" MELD points have been proposed for Budd-Chiari syndrome. A prospective validation is needed.

Selected Readings

Cazals-Hatem D, Vilgrain V, Genin P, et al. (2003) Arterial and portal circulation and parenchymal changes in Budd-Chiari syndrome: a study in 17 explanted livers. Hepatology 37:510–519

Durand F, Valla D (2005) Assessment of the prognosis of cirrhosis: Child-Pugh versus MELD. J Hepatol 42(Suppl):S100–107

Halff G, Todo S, Tzakis AG, et al. (1990) Liver transplanta-tion for the Budd-Chiari syndrome. Ann Surg 211:43–49.

Jamieson NV, Williams R, Calne RY (1991) Liver transplantation for Budd-Chiari syndrome, 1976–1990. Ann Chir 45:362–365

Langnas AN, Marujo WC, Stratta RJ, et al. (1992) A select-ive approach to preexisting portal vein thrombosis in patients undergoing liver transplantation. Am J Surg 163:132–136

Mahmoud AE, Helmy AS, Billingham L, Elias E (1997) Poor prognosis and limited therapeutic options in patients with Budd-Chiari syndrome and portal venous system thrombosis. Eur J Gastroenterol Hepatol 9:485–489

Mentha G, Giostra E, Majno PE, et al. (2006) Liver trans-plantation for Budd-Chiari syndrome: a European study on 248 patients from 51 centres. J Hepatol 44:520–528

Molmenti EP, Segev DL, Arepally A, et al. (2005) The utility of TIPS in the management of Budd-Chiari syndrome. Ann Surg 241:978–981; discussion 982–983

Murad SD, Valla DC, de Groen PC, et al. (2004) Determi-nants of survival and the effect of portosystemic shunting in patients with Budd-Chiari syndrome. Hepatology 39:500–508

Murad SD, Valla DC, de Groen PC, et al. (2006) Pathogenesis and treatment of Budd-Chiari syndrome combined with portal vein thrombo-sis. Am J Gastroenterol 101:83–90

Salvalaggio PR, Koffron AJ, Fryer JP, Abecassis MM (2005) Liver trans-plantation with simultaneous removal of an intracardiac transjugular intrahepatic portosystemic shunt and a vena cava filter without the utilization of cardiopulmonary bypass. Liver Transpl 11:229–232

Shaked A, Goldstein RM, Klintmalm GB, et al. (1992) Por-tosystemic shunt versus orthotopic liver transplantation for the Budd-Chiari syndrome. Surg Gynecol Obstet 174:453–459

Srinivasan P, Rela M, Prachalias A, et al. (2002) Liver transplantation for Budd-Chiari syndrome. Transplantation 73:973–977

Ulrich F, Steinmuller T, Lang M, et al. (2002) Liver transplantation in patients with advanced Budd-Chiari syndrome. Transplant Proc 34:2278

Valla DC (2003) The diagnosis and management of the Budd-Chiari syndrome: consensus and controversies. Hepatology 38:793–803

8
Liver Hemangioma

Alexis Laurent, Alain Luciani, and Daniel Cherqui

Pearls and Pitfalls

- Hemangioma is the most common benign liver tumor.
- Diagnosis is easy in most cases and relies on US for small lesions and MRI for large lesions.
- Most hemangiomas are asymptomatic and require no treatment.
- When present, symptoms include pain and discomfort and are related to the size of the lesion. Complications are very rare and include rupture, hemorrhage and consumptive coagulopathy.
- Indications for surgical resection are rare and include symptoms, complications or inability to exclude malignancy.
- Surgical techniques employed include enucleation and liver resection.
- When indicated, surgical intervention on these large lesions should be undertaken with caution and expertise since there is a risk of major intraoperative bleeding.

Introduction

Liver hemangioma (LH), also called cavernous hemangioma, is the most frequent benign liver lesion with a reported prevalence ranging between 1% and 10%. They are most

K.I. Bland et al. (eds.), *Liver and Biliary Surgery*,
DOI 10.1007/978-1-84996-429-6_8,
© Springer-Verlag London Limited 2011

commonly found in women, with a female/male ratio ranging from 3:1 to 5:1.

Pathology

LH are vascular tumors consisting of a cavity filled with blood. They have an unknown etiology although an association with estrogen therapy has been suggested. In 90% of the cases LH are solitary. They can be situated throughout the liver but classically are more often located in the right lobe.

The size of the lesions varies from a few millimeters to 30 cm or more. LH is referred to as "giant" when the size is greater than 10 cm. Lesions are well circumscribed and are often surrounded by a thin capsule. They can be seen at the surface of the liver but can rarely be pedunculated. In vivo, LH typically has a sponge consistency. When cut, the surface slice is red-brown and can include areas of hemorrhage or infarction.

Histologically, LH derives from the endothelial cells that line the blood vessels. They consist of multiple, large vascular channels lined by a single layer of endothelial cells and supported by collagenous walls. The vascular compartments are separated by thin fibrous septae and may contain thrombi. Large LH may develop a collagenous scar or fibrous nodule as thrombosis occurs. Rarely, stromal sclerosis may be associated with the absence of vascular cavities (sclerosing LH) and there may be focal stromal calcification.

Diagnosis and Natural History

While most LH remain small and asymptomatic, occasionally they may enlarge and give rise to various symptoms. When observed, 80% of LH remain stable in size, 15% grow slowly over a long period of time and less than 5% enlarge rapidly over a few months.

Most frequent symptoms include pain, discomfort or the occurrence of a palpable mass. All others causes of abdominal pain should be excluded before symptoms can be considered

to be related to LH. Pain can be due to capsular stretching, compression or displacement of surrounding structures or occurrence of a complication. Complications are very rare and include spontaneous rupture, intratumoral hemorrhage, thrombosis with infarction and consumptive coagulopathy (Kasabach-Merritt syndrome). Despite the high prevalence of LH, only about 30 cases of spontaneous rupture have been reported, which makes it an exceptional event.

Some studies have suggested that the lesion increases in size during pregnancy and estrogen therapy. It is for this reason that, as for adenoma, estrogen has been suggested to have a role in tumor growth.

Imaging

Typical LH usually present as asymptomatic incidentally discovered liver nodules on imaging studies, especially on ultrasonography (US). Typical US features are seen in small LH (<3 cm) and include the presence of a homogeneous well circumscribed hyperechoic lesion with subtle posterior acoustic enhancement (Fig. 8.1).

On CT scanning, hemangiomas usually disclose homogeneous hypodensity before injection. On dynamic contrast injections, lesions display early peripheral discontinuous, and progressive enhancement. On delayed phase imaging, the typical LH enhancement is complete (Fig. 8.2).

MRI is the most sensitive and specific imaging technique for LH identification, with sensitivity and specificity figures above 90%. The main MRI features of LH include the combination of a well circumscribed lobulated lesion, showing major hyper-intensity on T2 weighted images (Fig. 8.3). Following dynamic injection of gadolinium chelates, lesions behave similarly to CT with early peripheral, pseudo-nodular enhancement, leading to progressive and complete enhancement (Fig. 8.4). Combining T2 and post-injection features, the respective sensitivity and specificity of MRI for the diagnosis of LH reach 98% and 99%.

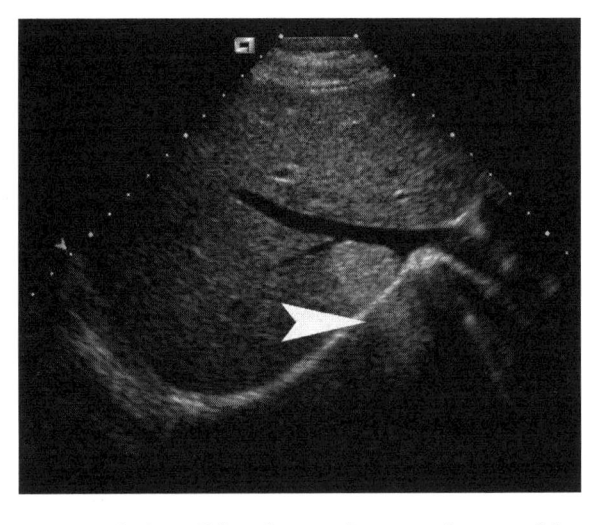

FIGURE 8.1. Typical small liver hemangioma on ultrasound: homogeneous well circumscribed hyperechoic with subtle posterior acoustic enhancement (arrow).

However, atypical imaging presentations are possible. Giant hemangiomas present on US as large heterogeneous masses. On CT and MR, such lesions exhibit early, peripheral, globular enhancement and on delayed phases, fail to demonstrate complete enhancement (> Fig. 8.5). Rapidly filling LH, whether on CT or on MRI, display a complete, intense enhancement beginning on arterial phase imaging, and persisting on portal and delayed phases of acquisition. A differential diagnosis with secondary endocrine lesions should be considered, but the persistent enhancement on delayed phases favors the diagnosis of LH. If calcification is present, this is usually situated peripherally. In this situation, definite diagnosis is rarely provided by imaging studies alone, as the normally observed high signal intensity of LH on MRI T2 weighted images can be hidden by the calcification. Sclerosing hemangiomas fail to show any of the characteristic features of LH and in particular lack their usual high signal intensity on T2 weighted images. Giant LH and rapidly filling LH and can by and large be diagnosed by specialized radiologists. The remaining atypical forms usually fail to be diagnosed confidently on imaging studies.

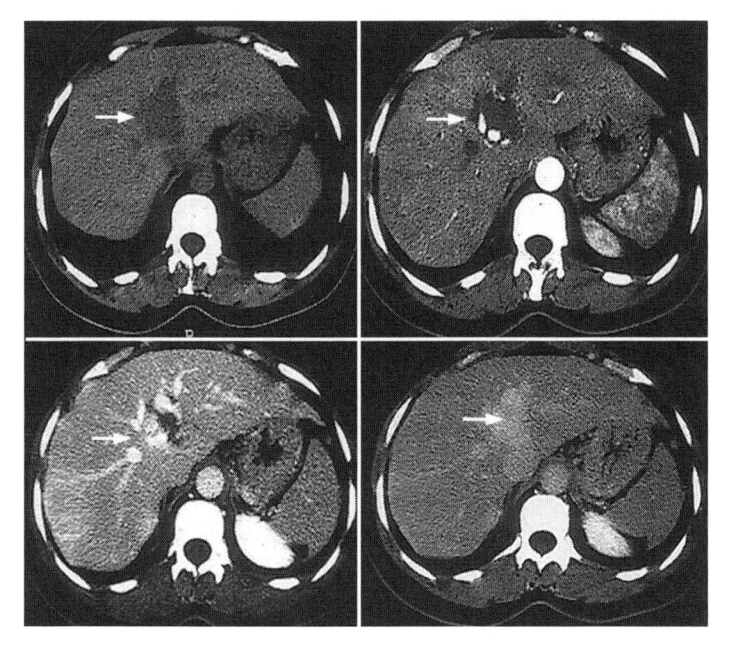

FIGURE 8.2. Typical liver hemangioma (arrowed) on CT: Hypodense lesion before contrast and centripedal filling after contrast with complete filling on delayed images.

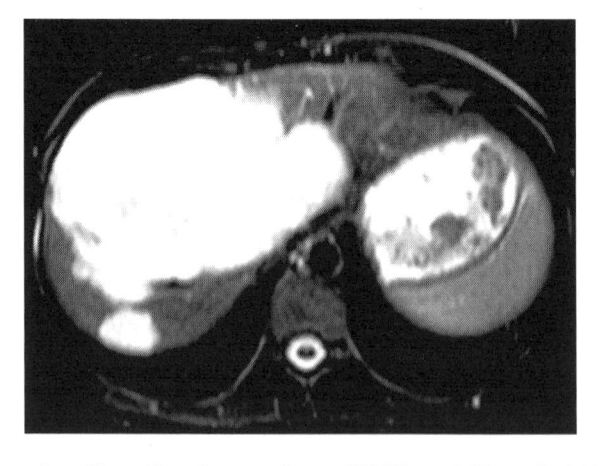

FIGURE 8.3. Giant liver hemangioma (GLH) on MR: typical highly hyperintense image on T2 weighted image.

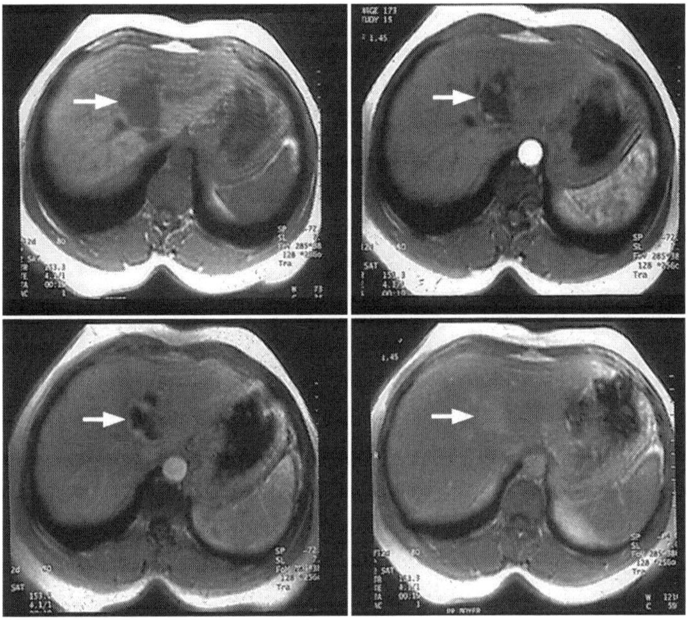

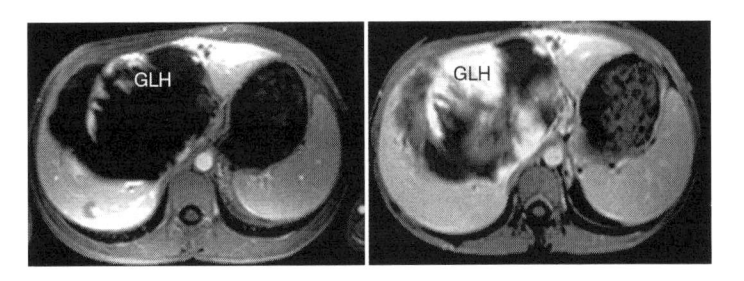

FIGURE 8.4. Typical liver hemangioma (arrowed) on MR: Hypointense T1 lesion before contrast and centripedal filling after contrast with complete filling on delayed images (same case as in Fig. 8.2).

FIGURE 8.5. Giant liver hemangioma (GLH) on MR: incomplete enhancement after IV contrast (same case as in Fig. 8.3).

Imaging diagnosis is possible in more than 90% of LH. In specific cases, however, a definite pathological diagnosis may be desirable, principally in patients with a history of cancer. Fine needle aspiration has been used but it can be dangerous

and has a low diagnostic yield. Surgical biopsy and frozen section during laparoscopy or laparotomy has been reported to have a better result and may avoid unnecessary resection.

Management

Once a diagnosis of LH has been established conservative management is the rule, because of their benign clinical course. Stability of the lesion should be established by repeated imaging at 3 months and at 1 year. Long term imaging surveillance is not justified when imaging is typical and the lesion is stable in size.

Cessation of estrogen therapy is controversial and only warranted in giant LH. Female patients should be informed of the possibility of growth in pregnancy. Radiotherapy and embolization have been proposed as a sole treatment or as a bridge to surgery but there are no data from reported series to substantiate this approach. Abscess formation has been reported following embolization. In exceptional cases of spontaneous rupture, emergency embolization prior to semi elective resection can be recommended.

There is no indication to consider resection of asymptomatic LH even when they are classified as giant. The only validated treatment is surgical resection but it is only indicated in three specific circumstances:

1. Giant LH with symptoms clearly related to the lesion
2. Complications of LH
3. Inability to exclude malignancy

Because only large and symptomatic LH should be resected, there is usually no place for a laparoscopic approach even although there has been an increasing trend in the use of this approach. Two types of resection technique can be considered. Some authors have described enucleation along the capsular plane since most LH are lined by a thin enclosing capsule. This is the procedure of choice when the capsular plane is easily found and it has been reported to be feasible in up to 60% of the cases. Temporary occlusion of the feeding arterial vessels may permit manual decompression of the

lesion and facilitate enucleation. In other situations, such as when no plane is found or there is doubt regarding underlying malignancy, formal liver resection is indicated. Since surgery may be difficult for giant LH, and can carry a substantial risk of bleeding, such interventions should be performed by experienced hepatic surgeons. In these cases, vascular clamping of the liver inflow and total vascular exclusion should be used liberally. Exceptionally, giant non resectable and highly symptomatic LH have required liver transplantation but only 3 such cases have been reported in the literature.

Conclusion

LH is the most frequent benign liver lesion but it is usually asymptomatic, follows a benign course, rarely enlarges and rarely gives rise to complication. Management of LH must follow strict rules (Fig. 8.6). Diagnosis must be obtained by good quality imaging including ultrasonography for small typical lesions and MRI for larger or atypical lesions. Asymptomatic patients with typical LH do not require treatment and can be

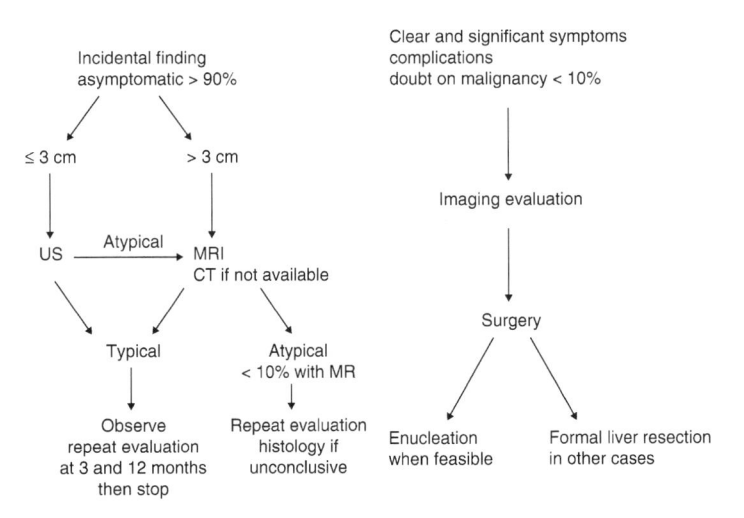

FIGURE 8.6. Liver hemangioma management algorithm.

safely observed, even if the lesion is large. Surgical resection should only be proposed for the rare symptomatic or complicated LH and parenchymal preserving procedures such as enucleation should be preferred. However, major liver surgery may occasionally be required.

Selected Readings

Baer HU, Dennison AR, Mouton W, et al. (1992) Enucleation of giant hemangiomas of the liver. Technical and pathologic aspects of a neglected procedure. Ann Surg 216:673–667

Corigliano N, Mercantini P, Amodio PM, et al. (2003) Hemoperitoneum from a spontaneous rupture of a giant hemangioma of the liver: report of a case. Surg Today 33:459–463

Farges O, Daradkeh S, Bismuth H (1995) Cavernous hem-angioma of the liver: are there any indications for resection? World J Surg 19:19–24

Gedaly R, Pomposelli JJ, Pomfret EA, et al. (1999) Cavernous hemangioma of the liver: anatomic resection vs. enu-cleation. Arch Surg 134:407–411

Gibney RG, Hendin AP, Cooperberg PL (1987) Sonographically detected hepatic hemangiomas: absence of change over time. Am J Roentgenol 149:953–957

Ishak KG, Rabin L (1975) Benign tumors of the liver. Med Clin North Am 59:995–1013

Motohara T, Semelka RC, Nagase L (2002) MR imaging of benign hepatic tumors. Magn Reson Imaging Clin N Am 10:1–14

Tepetes K, Selby R, Webb M, et al. (1995) Orthotopic liver transplantation for benign hepatic neoplasms. Arch Surg 130:153–156

Yamamoto T, Kawarada Y, Yano T, et al. (1991) Spontaneous rupture of hemangioma of the liver: treatment with trans-catheter hepatic arterial embolization. Am J Gastroenterol 86:1645–1649

Yoon SS, Charny CK, Fong Y, et al. (2003) Diagnosis, management and outcome of 115 patients with hepatic hem-angioma. J Am Coll Surg 197:392–402

Part II
Liver—Malignant

9
Hepatocellular Carcinoma

Sheung Tat Fan

Pearls and Pitfalls

- Hepatocellular carcinoma (HCC) is the third leading cause of cancer-related death among males.
- Hepatitis B and C infections are the etiologic cause in the majorityof patients.
- HCC is associated with a poor prognosis, because the tumor grows silently, spreads into luminal structures within the liver early, and being multicentric in origin, recurs frequently after the initial treatment.
- Planning of treatment depends on the extent of tumor spread, underlying liver function, remnant liver volume, and presence of concomitant medical disease.
- Liver transplantation and partial hepatectomy are effective treatment but are applicable in only 20% of patients. Combination therapy with radiofrequency ablation, transarterial chemoembolization, and/or intralesional alcohol injection together with close surveillance for recurrence are needed to attain long-term survival.
- Treatment of hepatitis B and C infection may reduce the incidence of HCC.
- Screening of high risk subjects, i.e. hepatitis B and C carriers, patients with cirrhosis, and family members of HCC, for detection of small tumors may improve the prognosis of HCC.

K.I. Bland et al. (eds.), *Liver and Biliary Surgery*,
DOI 10.1007/978-1-84996-429-6_9,
© Springer-Verlag London Limited 2011

Etiology

Hepatocellular carcinoma (HCC) is a highly lethal disease. It is the third leading cause of cancer-related death among males. The incidence is increasing rapidly in Western countries. Hepatitis B virus is the major etiologic factor in most countries in Asia and Africa. In contrast, hepatitis C virus is the most important cause in Japan, America, and Europe. Most of the patients with hepatitis B in Asia develop the infection in the neonatal period, yet it takes about 30–40 years before the hepatitis B virus produces pathologic changes of cirrhosis, which predisposes to development of HCC. Thus, the peak age for incidence of HCC is in the sixth decade. In contrast, younger patients with hepatitis B virus who have normal liver or chronic hepatitis may also develop HCC. The mechanism of formation of HCC may be different between patients with normal liver, chronic hepatitis, and cirrhosis. Smokers and alcoholics have a higher incidence of HCC if they are chronic hepatitis B carriers. Food contamination by aflatoxin and water contamination by microcystin may increase the risk of hepatitis B carriers to develop HCC. For hepatitis C, it takes about 30 years for cirrhosis and HCC to develop after the infection. Cirrhosis of other etiologies also predisposes to the development of HCC.

Pathology

Grossly, there are three macroscopic types of HCC. The massive type occurs in patients at a younger age with a non-cirrhotic liver. The neoplasms are large with adjoining "satellite" nodules which represent spread from the main neoplasm (Fig. 9.1). The cut surface is variegated due to necrosis and hemorrhage. The nodular type shows multiple grayish white, yellow, or brown nodules in a cirrhotic liver (Fig. 9.2). The diffuse type is the least common (Fig. 9.3), and grossly it may be indistinguishable from cirrhosis. Histologically, the liver is replaced by numerous small, disseminated tumor nodules. The disseminated type is missed frequently on imaging, but its presence should be suspected when major vessels are invaded.

- The presence of fluid outside the gallbladder fossa on ultrasound should not be dismissed as a normal post operative finding. In the presence of clinical signs or biochemical abnormalities, the detection of a fluid collection requires aspiration or drainage.
- Endoscopic stenting or sphincterotomy can be performed in the event of post operative bile leak and before referral of the patient to a specialist unit.
- A partial defect of the duct without tissue loss may be managed by primary closure with fine absorbable sutures without tension and with the use of sub hepatic drainage.
- A major duct injury requires reconstruction by a hepaticojejunostomy Roux-en-Y with a limb length of 70 cm between the biliary anastomosis and the entero-enterostomy. The anastomosis should be performed by a left duct approach using fine absorbable sutures, and a single layer anastomosis.
- The physical and psychological impact of bile duct injury is often underestimated.

Introduction

Laparoscopic cholecystectomy (LC) is one of the commonest general surgical operations carried out in the UK; 40,000 such procedures are carried out annually and laparoscopic cholecystectomy has, since the early 1990s, replaced open cholecystectomy as the surgical approach of choice. However, the adoption of the laparoscopic approach has resulted in an increased incidence of several previously recognized complications of open cholecystectomy, of which damage to the common bile duct (CBD) is the most serious with a reported incidence of approximately 0.5%. Bile duct injury (BDI) results in significant post operative mortality and morbidity and, even following a technically successful repair, often leads to reduced quality of life and long term survival. Bile duct injury is a particularly devastating complication given the favorable outcome and benign post operative course expected by both surgeon and patient prior to laparoscopic cholecystectomy, and this likely contributes to the large

13

Bile Duct Injury Following Laparoscopic Cholecystectomy

Stephen A. Boyce and O. James Garden

Pearls and Pitfalls

- Patients undergoing cholecystectomy should be informed of the risk of bile duct injury and the consequences of its occurrence.
- Careful dissection and correct interpretation of the biliary anatomy will avoid the complication of bile duct injury during cholecystectomy.
- The surgeon should understand that there is a reduction in the risk of injury when intra-operative cholangiogram is performed and earlier identification of bile duct injury but that its routine use does not eliminate the risk of bile duct injury.
- Conversion to open operation, cholecystostomy and subtotal cholecystectomy are all preferable to bile duct injury resulting from inappropriate attempts at removal of the gallbladder by laparoscopic means.
- Recognition of bile duct injury at the time of cholecystectomy requires immediate assistance or advice from an experienced hepatobiliary surgeon to enable assessment of its severity and the presence of a vascular injury, and to determine its appropriate management.
- Investigation for the possibility of bile duct injury should be undertaken in any patient who remains unwell in the 24 hours following apparently uneventful laparoscopic cholecystectomy.

K.I. Bland et al. (eds.), *Liver and Biliary Surgery*, DOI 10.1007/978-1-84996-429-6_13, © Springer-Verlag London Limited 2011

prudent when a prosthetic graft is being placed or if the patient has been unstable. The surgeon must use judgment and discretion to make a choice for each patient.

In contrast, patients with hemolytic anemia and gallstones, including sickle cell anemia, benefit clearly from prophylactic cholecystectomy when they undergo other abdominal operations, such as splenectomy. Patients with these diseases develop gallstones early in life and are likely to develop gallstone-related problems in the future. These patients have a clear indication for prophylactic cholecystectomy. Removal of gallbladders in obese patients who have already developed gallstones and undergo bariatric surgery is advocated by many surgeons. These patients frequently develop symptoms postoperatively, and symptoms may be difficult to separate from symptoms caused by complications of their primary operation. More controversial is removal of the gallbladder in obese patients without gallstones. Althoughstudies have documented a highrate of developing symptomatic gallstone disease within 6 months of operation during the period of maximal weight loss, it remains unclear whether the risk of cholecystectomy in all of these patients outweighs the benefit of prophylactic cholecystectomy, especially during a laparoscopic bariatric procedure.

Finally, some authors suggest that patientswith large gallstones (>2.5 cm), calcified gallbladders, and children are at increased risk to develop complications and might benefit from prophylactic cholecystectomy. Others consider prophylactic cholecystectomy for patients who will be traveling extensively or relocating to areas of the world with limited access to health care. In most cases, these indications require individualized plans with eachof the patients. Patients with spiculated, intramural gallbladder calcification ("porcelain gallbladder") are at increased risk of developing gallbladder cancer and should be considered strongly for gallbladder removal regardless of symptoms.

In summary, silent gallstones remain silent in the great majority of patients. The risk of observation versus cholecystectomyis either equal or slightly favors observation. Except in a few select patients, the great majorityof asymptomatic gallstones are best treated expectantly.

Selected Readings

Attili AF, DeSantis A, Capri R, et al. (1995) The natural history of gallstones: the GREPCO experience. Hepatology 21:656–660

Diehl AK (1991) Epidemiology and natural history of gallstone disease. Gastroenterol Clin N Am 20:1–19

Gracie WA, Ransohoff DF (1982) The natural history of silent gallstones. The innocent gallstone is not a myth. N EnglJMed 307:798–800

Hooper KD, Landis JR, Meilstrup JW, et al. (1991) The prevalence of asymptomatic gallstones in the general pop-ulation. Invest Rad 26:939–945

Juhasz ES, Wolff BG, Meagher AP, et al. (1994) Incidental cholecystectomy during colorectal surgery. Ann Surg 219:467–474

Kessaf A, Ertan T, Oguz H, et al. (2003) Impact of laparoscopy on frequency of surgery for treatment of gallstones. Surg Laparosc Endosc Percutan Tech 13:315–317

Klaus A, Hinder RA, Swain J, Achem SR (2002) Incidental cholecystectomy during laparoscopic antireflux surgery. Amer Surg 68:616–623

Meshikhes AW (2002) Asymptomatic gallstones in the laparoscopic era. JR Coll Surg Edin 47:742–748

Classification of Gallstone Disease by Clinical Presentation

Gallstones cause a wide spectrum of disease, ranging from no problems (asymptomatic gallstones) to potentially life-threatening complications such as perforated cholecystitis and gangrenous cholecystitis. Although most patients present with typical symptoms of postprandial pain (biliary colic), many patients have symptoms which mimic other upper gastrointestinal disorders, such as peptic ulcer or esophageal reflux disease. Other abdominal disorders may mimic symptoms of gallbladder disease. An understanding of the relationship between symptoms and gallstones is essential for studies examining the natural history of gallstones. For the purpose of this discussion, gallstones are best classified into three groups by clinical presentation.

Gallstones most often cause episodes of "biliary colic". Although termed colic, the pain is not colicky like intestinal or uterine colic. Rather, it is steady, severe, right upper quadrant or epigastric abdominal pain that may radiate into the back. These episodes of biliary colic occur as a crescendo/decrescendo pattern and last from 30 min to several hours in duration. Attacks begin 15–60 min after a meal (almost always the evening meal) and may be associated with nausea and, sometimes, bilious vomiting. Pain can be severe enough to bring the patient to the emergency department and require narcotic pain medication for relief. Patients report that episodes are often triggered by specific foods, including dairy products and fatty, fried, or spicy foods. Pain lasting more than 6 h suggests complicated gallstone disease (cholecystitis or pancreatitis) or another upper abdominal disorder. A patient presenting with a complication of gallstone disease, even if the complication was not preceded by episodes of biliary colic, is considered to have symptomatic gallstones and is at high risk for recurrent problems and requires treatment.

A second group of patients present with mild, vague symptoms consisting of mild transient pain, nausea, flatulence, and dyspepsia, often referred to as "non-specific" symptoms.

genetic predilection to gallstones; individuals with a family history of gallstones, and some ethnic groups such as American Indians, have a markedly increased chance of developing gallstones. In addition, obese men and women, especially during rapid weight loss, diabetic patients, patients with ileal disease or hemolytic anemia, and those treated with parenteral nutrition are at increased risk for developing gallstones.

Although prevalence of gallstones has not changed, our perspective on asymptomatic gallstones has changed greatly over the last 40 years. The magnitude and importance of asymptomatic gallstones became apparent as modern imaging modalities identified increasing numbers of patients with silent gallstones. Before the introduction of abdominal ultrasonography, physicians dealt almost exclusively with symptomatic individuals, and testing was not performed unless gallstones were clinically suspected. Oral cholecystography, which shows filling defects in a functioning gallbladder or non-visualization of the gallbladder on a double-dose test, was the imaging modality of choice; however, oral cholecystography was not and is not an appropriate test for wide-scale screening of patients.

Physicians developed a skewed perspective of gallstone disease and viewed it as a progressive disorder that rapidly and uniformly led to symptoms or complications. Complications of gallstones, such as acute or gangrenous cholecystitis, perforated cholecystitis, obstructive jaundice, and gallstone pancreatitis, were thought to occur frequently in untreated individuals and required emergent/urgent treatment increasing morbidity and mortality. The standard of care was operative intervention for all patients with gallstones, regardless of symptoms.

Abdominal ultrasonography, a reliable, non-invasive method of imaging gallstones, changed radically our concept of the development of gallstones and resultant, clinically important, gallstone disease. Asymptomatic gallstones, identified routinely in patients during examinations for other abdominal problems, were much more common than suspected previously. Moreover, ultrasonography provided a safe and effective means of following individuals with gallstones to determine their natural history.

Although gallstones may be the cause of these symptoms, they are just as likely to be caused by other gastrointestinal disorders, such as irritable bowel syndrome. Patients with mild symptoms, therefore, probably represent a diffuse group of disorders. Classically, they have poorer outcomes with cholecystectomy. Patients with these "non-specific" symptoms are best classified as mildly symptomatic patients and analyzed as a separate group in studies which examine the natural history of gallstones.

The final group of patients is of interest to this chapter. They are the truly asymptomatic patients. Their gallstones are identified incidentally during imaging performed for another problem or at operation during exploration. These patients deny symptoms attributable to gallstones and have never had a complication of gallstone disease.

The Natural History of Gallstones

Before discussing patients with asymptomatic gallstones, it is important to understand that patients with symptomatic gallstone are at risk to develop recurrent symptoms or complications. In the National Cooperative Gallstone Study, 69% of symptomatic patients experienced recurrent biliary colic within 2 years. McSherry et al. reported that 44% of symptomatic patients required biliary tract surgery within 6 years, while the GREPCO study showed that 6.5% of symptomatic patients developed serious complications of gallstone disease by 10 years. These studies remain the basis for recommending cholecystectomy to patients with symptoms attributed to gallstones, because patients are likely to continue to have episodes of pain and are at high risk to develop complications.

In contrast, the rate of conversion of silent to symptomatic gallstones is quite low. This was first recognized and documented by Gracie and Ransohoff in 1982 who studied 123 faculty members (mostly male) with silent gallstones at the University of Michigan. Conversion to symptomatic disease occurred in only 10% of patients by 5 years, 15% by 10 years,

and 18% by 15 years. The study was criticized, however, because it might not apply to women who more commonly develop gallstones, but subsequent studies including large numbers of women revealed that only about 1–2% of asymptomatic patients develop symptoms per year, and another 1–2% per year developed complications, an acceptably low rate. The majority of patients do not require operation for as long as 20 years, and several studies show that the rate of developing symptoms and complications decrease after 10–15 years.

Patients with mild symptoms fall into an intermediate category requiring operation more frequently than asymptomatic patients (6–8% per year); however, the rate of serious complications in these patients is low, about 1–3% of patients per year. Mildly symptomatic patients act more like asymptomatic patients than symptomatic patients.

General Recommendations for Patients with Asymptomatic Gallstones

Patients with asymptomatic gallstones develop symptoms infrequently, and the majority remain asymptomatic for long periods of time. Serious complications, such as acute cholecystitis or gallstone pancreatitis, occur at acceptably low rates of about 1–2% of patients per year. Currently, treatment of patients with complications is almost as safe as elective operation. Risk analysis, using the data accumulated on the natural history of gallstones and the current rates of morbidity and mortality for cholecystectomy, estimates that observation of patients with asymptomatic gallstones has a risk less than or equal to operation. When faced with equal risk, most patients will choose observation. The current recommendation is that asymptomatic gallstones be treated expectantly. Cholecystectomy is, with some exceptions discussed later, reserved for patients who develop symptoms or complications. Consideration of gallbladder cancer does not change recommendations; gallbladder cancer develops in less than 1 (gallstone) patient per 1,000 per year. Analysis of cost effectiveness and life expectancy support

this recommendation, showing no advantage of prophylactic cholecystectomy over observation. It is not surprising that operation on patients who do not have symptoms does not improve the health-related quality of life as it does for asymptomatic patients.

Mildly symptomatic gallstone patients are also generally not candidates for cholecystectomy. If symptoms increase in frequency or interfere with lifestyle, and the patient understands the distinct possibility that cholecystectomy may not resolve the problems, cholecystectomy may be considered.

Prophylactic Cholecystectomy

Select groups of patients with asymptomatic gallstones may be at increased risk of developing symptoms or complications warranting prophylactic cholecystectomy, depending on their level of risk. In the past, prophylactic cholecystectomy was recommended for diabetic patients with silent gallstones, because they had a higher incidence of gallstones, greater risk of complications, and increased morbidity and mortality for emergent or urgent operation. Recent studies addressed this issue by documenting that only about 15% of diabetic patients with asymptomatic gallstones developed symptoms by 5 years compared with 48% of diabetic patients with symptoms These results are comparable to non-diabetic patients. More importantly, the morbidity and mortality of biliary tract operations on diabetic patients were similar or only slightly higher than those performed on nondiabetic patients. Like non-diabetic patients, the risks and benefits of operation versus observation are similar, and prophylactic cholecystectomy in diabetic patients with asymptomatic gallstones is no longer recommended. Although some have advocated prophylactic cholecystectomy for organ transplant patients (many of whom are diabetic), citing the potential for increased morbidity and mortality when the patient is immunosuppressed, current data indicates that these patients are also most optimally treated expectantly.

Cirrhotic patients have an increased incidence of gallstones, and biliary tract surgeryis associated with greater morbidity and mortality in these patients. Therefore, controversy exists concerning treatment of both symptomatic and asymptomatic cirrhotic patients. Twenty-three of 58 cirrhotic patients with gallstones were observed and did not develop symptoms. The morbidity and mortality in those patients who underwent cholecystectomy were acceptable in Child A and B patients, although all patients required blood transfusion, a rare event in non-cirrhotic patients. Ten percent of Child C patients died, and 40% developed clinically important complications. In another study, 82% of cirrhotic patients with asymptomatic gallstones remained symptom-free, and only six patients developed acute cholecystitis or pancreatitis. In summary, cirrhotic patients with gallstones develop symptoms infrequently and can be treated safely once symptoms develop in Child A or B patients. Careful observation with silent stones is reasonable, but because Child C patients experience high operative morbidity and mortality, early intervention is warranted once symptoms appear in Child A and B patients.

Treatment of asymptomatic gallstones found before or during abdominal operation performed for another reason, remains controversial. Very little data are available to guide surgeons for most operations. Removal of the gallbladder in 195 gallstone patients undergoing a primary colon operation did not add morbidity or mortality to the colectomy. In comparison, of the 110 patients in the same study who did not undergo prophylactic cholecystectomy, symptoms requiring cholecystectomy developed in 12% by 2 years and 22% by 5 years. Considering the high incidence of developing symptomatic gallstones postoperatively, and the low morbidity and mortality of the added procedure, prophylactic cholecystectomy is reasonable, unless otherwise contraindicated during elective colonic operations. Likewise, cholecystectomy has been studied during laparoscopic antireflux operations and did not increase the morbidity or mortality of the primary operation. Extrapolating these data to other abdominal operations appears logical, if the primary operation is proceeding without problem, and the patient's condition allows for additional anesthetic time. It may not be